ΔD A ⌐⌐⌐ign

The Tragic in Architecture

Guest-edited by Richard Patterson

Ⓦ WILEY-ACADEMY

Architectural Design
Vol 70 No 5 October 2000

ISBN 0-471-89274-2
Profile No 147

Editorial Offices
International House
Ealing Broadway Centre
London W5 5DB
T: +44 (0)20 8326 3800
F: +44 (0)20 8326 3801

Editor
Maggie Toy

Managing Editor
Helen Castle

Production
Mariangela Palazzi-Williams

Art Director
Christian Küsters ↘ CHK Design

Design Assistant
Owen Peyton Jones ↘ CHK Design

Advertisement Sales
01243 843272

Photo Credits
∆ Architectural Design

Abbreviated positions
b=bottom, c=centre, l=left, t=top

P 4 courtesy Foster and Partners, photo: Nigel Young; p 6 © Richard Patterson; p 8 © National Gallery, London; p 9(t) © National Gallery, London; p 9 (b) courtesy Robert Maxwell; p 10 courtesy Robert Maxwell; p 11 © Louvre, Paris, France/Peter Willi/Bridgeman Art Library; p 13 courtesy Robert Maxwell; p 14 courtesy Robert Maxwell; pp 16, 18, 20, 22 and 23 courtesy John Outram Associates, © John Outram; p 24 © Architectural Association/FR Yerbury; p 26 © Charles Jencks; p 28 © Architectural Association/Valerie Bennett; pp 30–31, 32, 33, 34 (tl) and 34 (tl) courtesy Foster and Partners, photo: Nigel Young; 34 (tr) © Richard Davies; pp 37, 39, 40, 41, 42 and 43 courtesy Richard Patterson; pp 44–46, 47 (t), 47 (b), 49, 50 and 51 courtesy David Chipperfield Architects, © David Chipperfield Architects; p 47 (c) courtesy David Chipperfield Architects, © Richard Davies; p 54 and 57 © Pei Cobb Freed Architects; p 55, p 56 (tl), p 56 (c), p 56 (b), p 58 (b) and p 59 © Timothy Hursley; p 56 (tr) courtesy of USHMM Photo Archives, photo: Max Reid; p 58 (tl) courtesy of USHMM Photo Archives, photo: Beth Redlich; p 58 (tr) courtesy of USHMM Photo Archives, photo: Edward Owen; p 60, 63 and 64 © Eisenman Architects; p 61 © Richard Patterson; p 62 courtesy Ute Hejmrod Architecture and Culture Management, Berlin, photo: © Robert Kruse; pp 66–67, 68, 71, 72, 73, 74 and 75; p 76 © Yael Padan; p 78 courtesy Ram Karmi Architects, photos (tl, tr, b): Tal Levi-Karmi; p 78 (c) © Duby Tal & Moni Haramati – Albatross; p 80 (tl), (tc) and (tr) © Yael Padan; p 80 (cl), (cr), (bl) and (br) Guggenheim/Bloch Architects and Urbanists photos: Yoram Leheman; p 82 and 85 © Julie Cook; p 86 (t) courtesy Jay Joplin (London); p 86 © Edward Winters; p 88, 90 and 91 © Jane Hamlem.

∆+
P 95+ (t) courtesy Françoise-Hélène Jourda; p 95+ Palais de Justice and Academy of Further Education photos: courtesy Françoise-Hélène Jourda, © Paul Raftery; p 95+(cl) and (2nd b) School of Architecture, Lyon: courtesy Françoise-Hélène Jourda, photo by Georges Fessy; p 95+(cr) School of Architecture, Lyon: courtesy Françoise-Hélène Jourda, photo by S Couturier; p 96+ (t) courtesy Odile Decq; p 96+ photos of installation and Banque Populaire: courtesy Odile Decq, photos by Georges Fessy; p 96+ all courtesy Manuelle Gautrand, © Philippe Ruault; pp 98+, 99+, 100+ and 101+ courtesy Martin Pearce, Portsmouth University School of Architecture; p 98+ (l) courtesy Haig Beck; 102+, 103+, 104+ and 105+ © Thomas Deckker; pp 106+, 107+, 108+ and 109+ © General, Lighting and Power; p 112+ © Strasman Architects Inc.

Cover: photo © Hélène Binet.

Subscription Offices UK
John Wiley & Sons Ltd.
Journals Administration Department
1 Oaklands Way, Bognor Regis
West Sussex, PO22 9SA
T: +44 (0)1243 843272
F: +44 (0)1243 843232
E: cs-journals@wiley.co.uk

Subscription Offices USA and Canada
John Wiley & Sons Ltd.
Journals Administration Department
605 Third Avenue
New York, NY 10158
T: +1 212 850 6645
F: +1 212 850 6021
E: subinfo@wiley.com

Annual Subscription Rates 2000
Institutional Rate: UK £135
Personal Rate: UK £90
Student Rate: UK £60
Institutional Rate: US $225
Personal Rate: US $145
Student Rate: US $105

∆ is published bi-monthly.
Prices are for six issues and include postage and handling charges. Periodicals postage paid at Jamaica, NY 11431. Air freight and mailing in the USA by Publications Expediting Services Inc, 200 Meacham Avenue, Eimont, NY 11003

Single Issues UK: £19.99
Single Issues outside UK: US $32.50
Order two or more titles and postage is free. For orders of one title ad £2.00/US $5.00. To receive order by air please add £5.50/US $10.00

Postmaster
Send address changes to ∆ c/o Expediting Services Inc, 200 Meacham Avenue, Long Island, NY 11003

Printed in Italy. All prices are subject to change without notice.
[ISSN: 0003-8504]

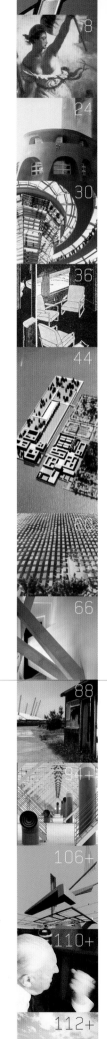

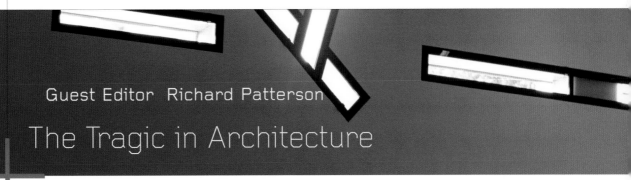

Guest Editor Richard Patterson

The Tragic in Architecture

ΛD   Architectural Design +

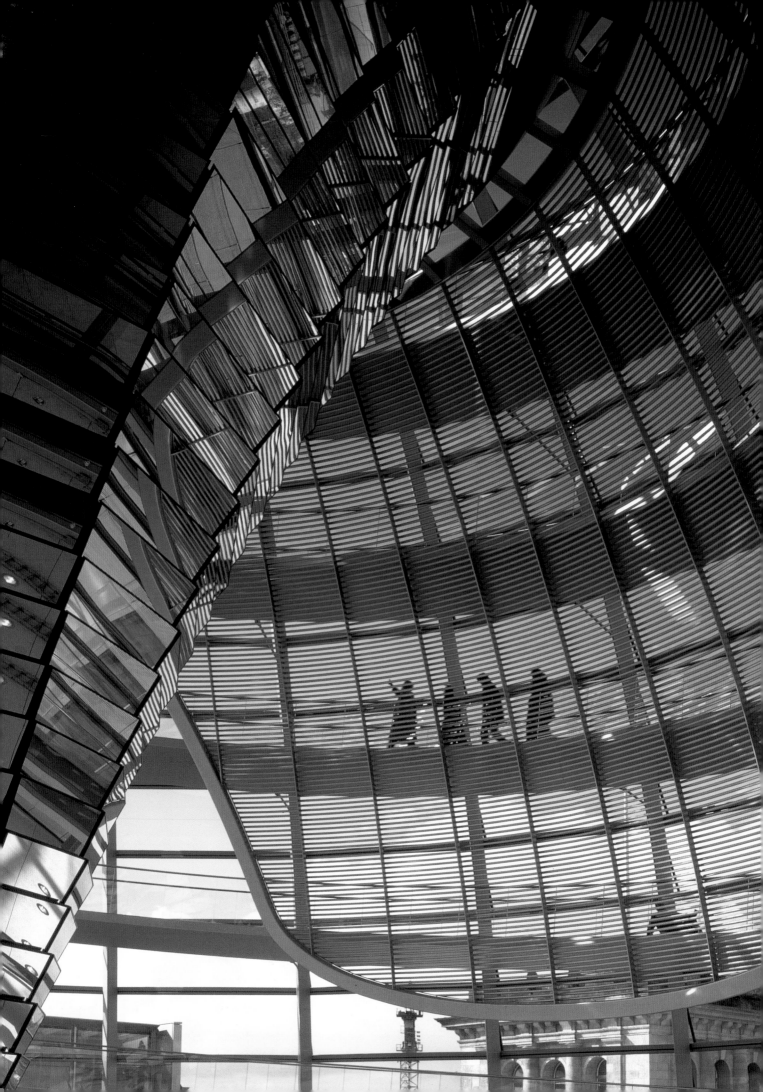

At a time when the popular conception of tragedy lies somewhere between traditional literary pathos, the personal revelations that dominate 'the confessional' culture of the media and the Beegees screeching at the tops of their voices, the tragic is a brave theme for $\triangle$ to embark on. For rather than exclusively exploring buildings that commemorate or express human 'tragedies', this title investigates the potential of tragedy as a genre in architecture. A genre that is classical in origin and has been more deeply rooted in literature than the visual arts. This could all be regarded as profoundly unfashionable. For any discussion of the tragic positions itself outside the more narcissistic contemporary obsessions with speed and surface appearance, which have in recent years intensified with the exponential growth of new media. This title demands a broader perspective of modern architecture, as it places often monumental contemporary buildings in a much wider historical context: a context that is concerned with significance and cultural thought over form and style. This is, for the present climate, a rare and daring exploration into architecture's meaning.

As Richard Patterson explains, somewhat modestly, in his own introduction, 'The Tragic in Art and Architecture' was originally the subject of a symposium organised by Wiley-Academy, the publishers of *Architectural Design*. Only two of the contributions published here – Robert Maxwell's opening essay and Patterson's text 'The Metamorphosis of Tragedy' – were the basis of talks given at the Royal Academy. Since the event in the Spring of 1999, Patterson has intently developed the title as a theme. The result is not only that he has introduced an almost entirely new cast to participate in the publication, but that his thesis has shifted and matured from the one that was originally proposed. In so doing, he has also ensured that he has covered, with his section on the Holocaust, the most serious and conspicuous example of tragedy as a human theme in the 20th century. This is not at the total expense of the everyday and the unexpected. For the issue closes with contributors seeking out the tragic in places as diverse as Soho's Colony Club, Tracey Emin's Bed and the notorious Millennium Dome. $\triangle$

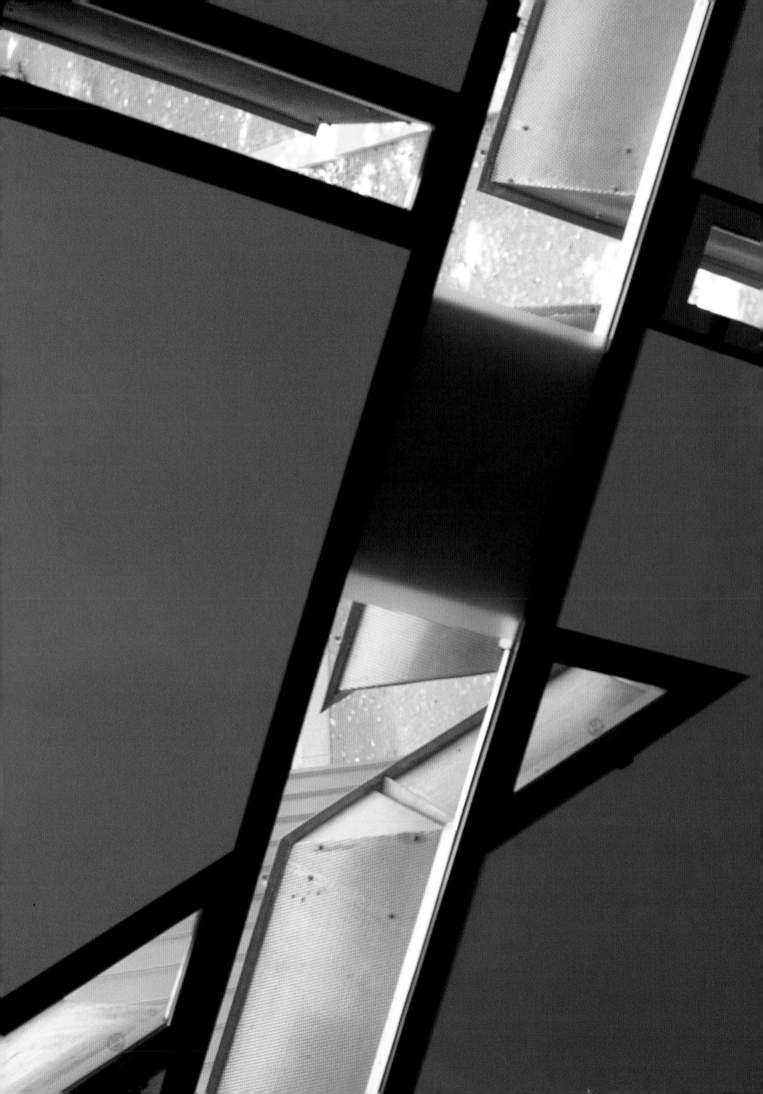

This issue of Ɒ follows on from the symposium, 'The Tragic in Art and Architecture', initiated by Jeremy Melvin and Robert Maxwell and held at the Royal Academy in March 1999. It explored the possibility of the 'tragic' as an extreme form of representation and narrative in architecture and other visual art forms. The terms 'narrative' and 'tragedy' can vary greatly in meaning, and this is reflected in the breadth of positions and assumptions adopted by the various contributors here.

The notion that architecture can convey a message, however vague, is based on the presumption that it is structured like a written text that can in some way be 'read' as a narrative and is capable of sustaining a reflective and critical analysis of events or of portraying explicit meanings. The iconographic tradition, particularly of the 16th to the 18th centuries, would be a case in point, but even this was based on images expressed only through painting and sculpture. Vitruvius' discussion of appropriate styles of architecture (Doric, Ionic or Corinthian) provided the grounds for an attempt to justify belief in an aesthetic naturalism: that architectural form and decoration have a natural propriety and meaning. But in addition to its potential textual coherence, architecture provides a site and a framework within which narratives of independent origin come to be registered and judged.

The argument presented in this issue begins properly with Renaissance classical architecture. As historians have long known, the architecture of the Renaissance was not a historical or archaeological revival of Rome. It was a new invention, based on an odd collection of material fragments of old buildings, stitched together by Alberti into a theoretical, systematic whole, by way of compositional principles and values derived from elsewhere. If we inspect those principles, we discover that they are largely derived, as in Vitruvius, from rhetoric, and moreover, from principles that have their origin in tragedy.

Classical 'imitation' can be either imitation of an 'idea' or of another imitation. In the case of a painting, the imitation is of another image; in the drawing of geometric forms, the imitation is of an idea. In the case of architecture, imitation is of a type, motif or figure, possibly metaphorically, of nature, but given that architecture is not natural, always of an abstract idea. In the classical world (prior to Neoclassical academic architecture) the execution of architecture was never by way of direct copy, but always by way of emulation. It was an imitation, but not of the world of appearances.

To Aristotle, 'tragedy is essentially an imitation not of persons but of action and life, happiness and misery'. 'Imitation' in the sense that Aristotle used it is emphatically not a synonym for replication. The tragic, in imitating events, leaves out a substantial amount of 'realistic' detail. Tragedy is not, in fact, a representation of the world as it actually is. It is, rather, a genre, in which certain events or actions are presented in terms of their significance for a particular subject over a limited period of time.

In the essays that follow, the question of the expressive capability of architecture is explored in many different ways. In some areas, it is the formal legacy that is of central concern. In others, there is greater emphasis on the expression of what at various times has been referred to as 'tragic': the experience and observation of fear and pity. Ɒ

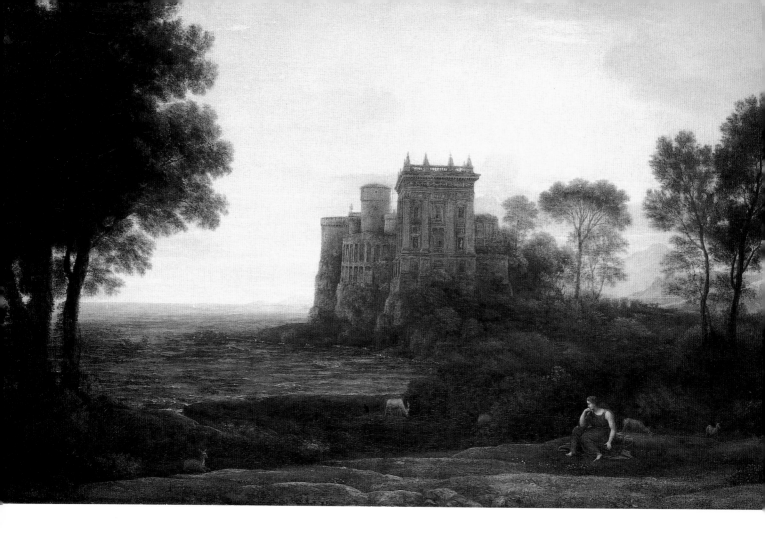

Approaching the Void:
Can the Tragic appear in Architecture?

The view that architecture can still aspire to heroic grandeur as a framework for the tragic becomes progressively more uncertain in modern times. Rather than proclaiming the propriety of the civic, collective and social, the culture of the West has become a critical system of enquiry. However, Robert Maxwell attests to the possibility of a communication of the tragic in the midst of this instability of signifiers.

The contemporary fascination with Minimalism can be regarded as an attempt to explore the limits of expression.[1] By eliminating almost everything, by leaving almost nothing, could we begin to sense what are the essentials? This has parallels with the theme of the tragic. Can art approach the unspeakable? Can it engender a sense of the limits of life and human understanding? Can it approach the tragic? And if art can do so, can architecture do so too?

The tragic demands death, the event from which there is no going back. But it is not simply the fact of death, but its impact in a defined poetic context. The multiplication of death does not induce the tragic. The Black Death, the potato famine, the daily earthquake, are simply calamities. The 'tragic death' of baby William, shaken to death by his au pair, is sad indeed, but not by itself tragic. Tragedy and comedy are genres, initially of the theatre. They follow a certain form, adumbrate a set of rules, and require the participation of an audience. Greek tragedy required the death of the Hero. Medieval tragedy celebrated the death of the Saviour. Renaissance tragedy brought back the hero, not as myth, but as one of us, the simply human.

The staging of tragedy requires artifice. It must follow a narrative protocol. It stipulates a rhetorical skill, like Shakespeare's abundant skill as a playwright, and Elizabethan tragedy is still effective for us. In 1961, George Steiner claimed that we had already witnessed the *Death of Tragedy*, in his book of that name, because poetic language no longer holds the central position it did in the times of Dante and Shakespeare. But where language has lost other forms of expression have gained, and tragedy can be staged today in new and different ways. The random spills of earth around the grave-like setting of Pina Bausch's *Viktor* (1986), for example, are banal and repetitive events that in context take on a deeper meaning and open the door to the tragic sense, expressed through dance. Without words, expression of the absurdity of life is accompanied by renewal of compassion.

The tragic abounds in all traditional art that starts from grandeur. It deals with figures choreographed so as to create a narrative, for which the title is often an essential script. The heroic event was the culminating *theme* of all serious painting, and was still clearly alive with Nicolas Poussin and not too distant in Claude Lorrain. But in both we sense a diminution of belief, a surge of the merely aesthetic. Can the tragic survive this loss of belief?

If architecture, whose tropes are unspoken, cannot so clearly evoke a heroic past, it has still been associated with the heroic scale of values. Architecture provided the framework for the epic sculptures placed in the pediments of the Greek temples. It was admitted not for itself, but for the setting it provided, by which the sacred could be made accessible and approached by ordinary people. We can argue that this role, at least, is still open to it today.

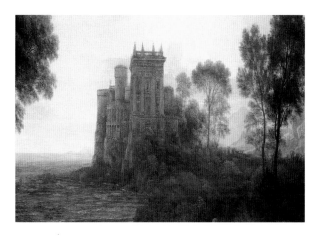

With Claude, architecture acquires an expressive presence, linking it to the heroic event enacted in the foreground. In his *Landscape with Psyche and the Palace of Love* (1664), he willingly incorporates the building type of the palace into the fable. Similarly, in the construction of the social world, architecture became an essential channel through which myth could enter daily life. During the Baroque, it was expected to confer *gravitas* where needed, and it is easy to recognise this in Francesco Borromini, his San Carlo alle Quattro Fontane of 1637–41 for example.

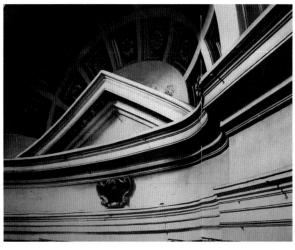

In such an example, we cannot claim that the tragic is directly expressed, rather that in mediating the worship of the hero-redeemer the building partakes of the tragic. Without it, the mystery of faith could not enter ordinary life.

Opposite
Claude Lorrain, *Landscape with Psyche and the Palace of Love*, National Gallery, London, 1664.

Right
Francesco Borromini, S Carlo alle Quattro Fontane, Rome (detail of cornice) 1637–41.

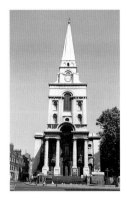

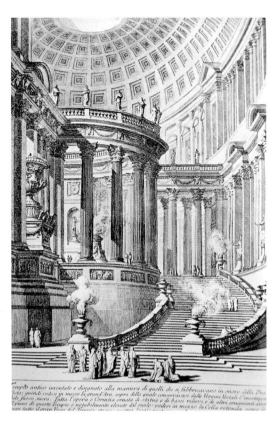

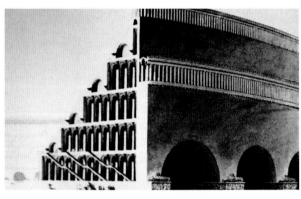

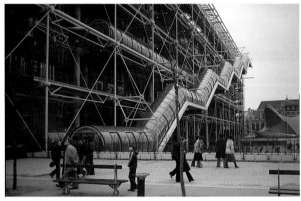

After the *terribilitá* evoked in Mannerism, the Baroque is more closely linked to matters of faith – the whole trauma of the Counter-Reformation. Yet one senses very little faith in the somewhat political programme of building city churches during the time of Christopher Wren and Nicholas Hawksmoor, and the return of a subdued sense of the terrible in Hawksmoor seems to have more to do with the autonomy of architecture, with freely rearranging its syntax, evolved for a sacred purpose no doubt, but now concerned with exploring more abstract possibilities.

With Piranesi, one can make more of a case that the original drawings do indeed express a feeling in their own right, a feeling close to a sense of the destiny of man and his frailty. For Piranesi, the building was an essential means by which to approach high emotions. He had an eye for ruins, and the ancient world lay all about him in ruins. To depict the fall of architecture came close to depicting the fall of man. And even when he constructed a fictive world, as with his fantasy on the Temple of Vesta (1762), we sense the limits of attainment, the arbitrariness of design, the hubris of man who now appears dwarfed by his own creations.

Étienne-Louis Boullée (1728–99) shrinks man to even tinier dimensions, so that in a world of heroic stature, he is of no more significance than an ant. His *Intérieur d'un Cirque 1er projet*, with its escape stairs shown in abstract section, is like an anticipation of the Pompidou Centre: it reduces man to part of a crowd. All grandeur has been absorbed by the building.

The decline of heroic status was already implied in the 18th-century search for the sublime, where man is confronted by the limits beyond which nature is indifferent to his destiny. On the one hand, the heroic becomes visible as a fiction; on the other, nature becomes visible as a machine. The machine aesthetic, insofar as it denies humanity and prefers a studied indifference, raises a certain pathos, even if it does not quite touch the sublime. With the Romantics, this indifference has undermined belief and generated a new sense that man is alone.

Delacroix's *Liberty Leading the People* (1830) is a figure of rhetoric, an abstraction made vivid by the use of the female form. Man is free, but he has no witness; unless it is the architecture that now provides that witness, reflecting as it does the weight of society, marking the action with its indisputable evidence of time and place. Here, social justice replaces theological retribution.

And as the metaphysical limits of art itself became visible, around the time of the First World War, art returned to the theme of the building as witness, now reinforced by architecture's capacity to represent not only reality but, through its recurrence in dreams, becoming even a kind of surrogate conscience or

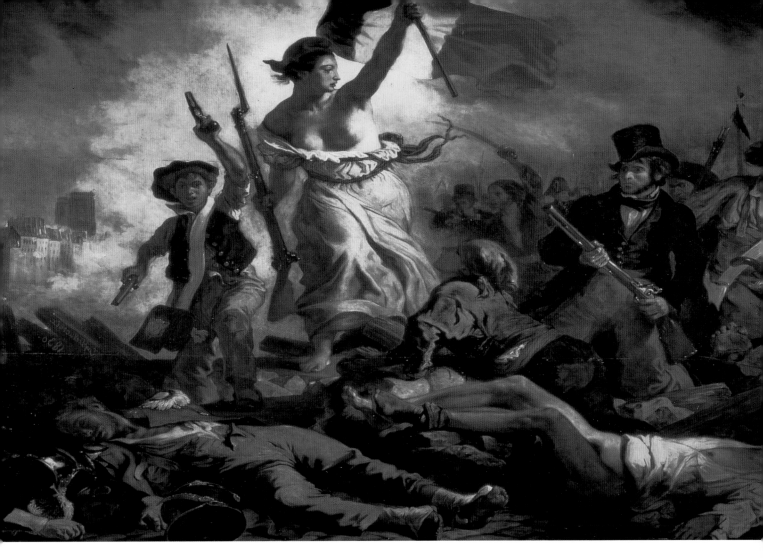

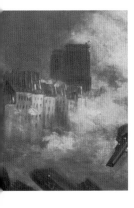

embodiment of memory. Practically all of Giorgio de Chirico's 'metaphysical' art is the direct expression of this malaise.

But this demands that art exercise a capacity for representation, and it is notorious that Aldo Rossi's contribution to the Postmodern movement of the 1970s is broadly based on De Chirico's use of representation. However, both abstraction and conceptual thought, the over riding discoveries of 20th-century art, have cast a doubt over representation, substituting the art object as itself the final mystery of life. Abstract art transfers attention from object-as-means to object-as-end. The art object no longer offers itself as a window on to life, but directly engages our cognitive faculties. By becoming an enigma, it resists being emptied of meaning. In Abstract Expressionism, the meaning is smothered by personal expressionism – personal expression. Instead of meaning, we have meaningfulness. With Franz Kline, with Robert Motherwell, we accede to the power of the gesture, but we still obstinately attempt to animate the figure. We search the gesture for a meaning, taking the title as clue, as script of a lost narrative. And indeed, each form embodies a strong character that stirs ambiguous associations and stimulates the imagination. The very name Abstract Expressionism suggests that something be expressed, that some content has survived.

I was much struck by Sean Scully's recent review of a Mark Rothko retrospective.[2] Scully, who is an artist as well as a critic, denies that abstraction supplants all figurative content, and insists that Rothko's severe rectangles still constitute figures. As figures, they are receptive to the projections we can bring to them, and they are nothing if not emotive. The critic Richard Cork has said: 'We cannot help seeing in these great veils of orange, red, black, yellow or maroon a host of possible references to the visible world.'

Rothko seems to be a special case, even for devotees of pure aesthetics. He is among those abstractionists, including Agnes Martin, whose very restricted system insinuates a moral stance. His early paintings were more figurative, and the ever-increasing austerity throughout his life suggests renunciation. The word 'tragic' has been applied to his work, without referring particularly to the coincidence of the final black works and his subsequent suicide.

Francis Bacon, in his interviews with David Sylvester (1975–80), spoke of a method of portraiture that seeks to isolate the subject as a sort of event staged within a frame. The background is clean, elegant, complete; in context, the smeared paint on the face, the distortion of the figure, take on a suggestion of movement, of something glimpsed rather than seen. This is analogous to the method by which Heidegger deals with essence as being no longer something that can be fully grasped, but something that still leaves a kind of cultural trace. By metaphoric extension, this sense of a fugitive presence, through Bacon's magic, succeeds in communicating an impression of life and pain. What he wanted to do, he said, was to isolate the image and take it away from the interior and the home.

In espousing this ambition, Bacon sets up a dialectic in which the interior and the home are seen as private and makeshift, and a public realm emerges that is identified with something inescapable, like a judgement and a destiny. He evidently wants to reinstate a sense of the human condition defined by loss and pain. His use of triptychs in a secular situation signals that the mystery has stepped down from the altar and invaded private life. This is surely close to a tragic view of life. It is, of course, an interesting paradox that many of the settings depict the interior and the home in lurid terms, showing the horror encountered in bedrooms and bathrooms, and the desperation that assails the individual at his most naked and vulnerable.

a photograph would have done. In both cases, the change of style acts as a framing device to intensify the meaning.

Within architecture in the course of the 20th century, abstract forms have triumphed at the expense of symbolic resonance. With the loss of the classical orders, there is no upstanding metaphor for the human figure; a fact that gives peculiar interest to John Outram's invention of the 'robot order' made from service ducts. With the literal interpretation of functionality, architecture is reduced to utility, deprived of expression, expected to reveal nothing but the physical trace of human movement. The 'machine for living' places a particular stress on the ergonomic aspects which literally fit the body, such as the mechanisms of bathroom and kitchen, staircase and ramp. These took exemplary form with Le Corbusier's Villa Savoye (1929–31). In museums, the same approach can result in a complete complex of ramps, escalators, elevators and staircases, conduits and outlets, comprising a total life-support system more

The 'machine for living' places a particular stress on the ergonomic aspects which literally fit the body, such as the mechanisms of bathroom and kitchen, staircase and ramp.

Bacon uses a combination of abstraction and figuration – and we must acknowledge that there is nothing in art theory to deny this method. The difference between the two modes acts as a framing device, suggesting two different levels of existence. In the 'staging' of meaning, particular advantage may be taken of a combination of both. Where realism tends to kill the life it depicts (as with Soviet Socialist Realism) a measure of abstraction, by stepping back from life, may suggest life more vividly.

Kasimir Malevich's famous image of Suprematist architecture montaged on to a photograph of New York (1923) suggests the displacement of the old by the new, in an opposition where the new is accorded the advantage of artistic expression so that it can speak for the future. Similarly, in Adolphe Mouron Cassandre's poster for the Nord Express (1927), the abstracted handling of the locomotive's mechanism, privileged as art, suggests actual movement more vividly than

appropriate to the conquest of space than to exploration of culture. The Archigram idea assumed that the resources available for the military exploration of space should be appropriated for the enjoyment of ordinary citizens. The service system as art object here assumes transcendental importance, and nothing is left of the privilege that Aristotle assigned to architecture: to provide the site where fine art may celebrate the sacred myths.

In its most extreme form as a mere servant – the shopping mall – architecture has no voice of its own. Management of the mall includes management of its architecture. But oddly, life attains its own momentum, no matter into what receptacle it is poured. The High-tech atrium has become so widely imitated that it now means no more than that the developer wants to be in the swim. The atrium, pioneered at the Eaton Center in Toronto (1977), has become a commonplace of shopping malls, indeed, of public buildings. As a functional device, its aim is not to uplift the spirit but to provide the pleasurable sensations that encourage retail sales. If this precludes the tragic, as it must

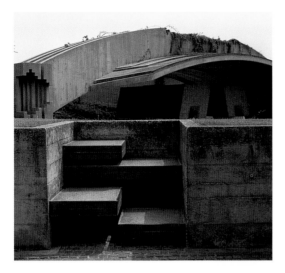

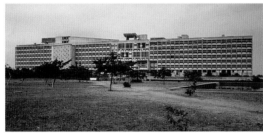

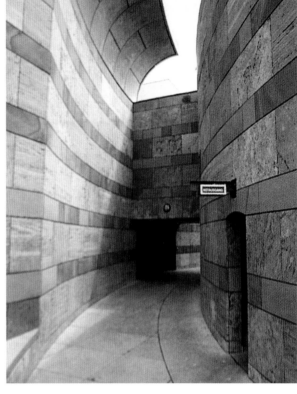

Top left
Carlo Scarpa, Brion-Vega
cemetery, San Vito d'Avitole,
Treviso, 1970–2.

Bottom left
Le Corbusier, United Nations
Secretariat building at
Chandigarh, 1947.

Right
James Stirling, Staatsgalerie,
Stuttgart, 1977–84.

surely do, it is hardly surprising. If the overwhelming totality of functional architecture is dedicated to an everyday banality, it can hardly be expected to rise to a higher plane of expression. Yet today, after Frank Gehry's Bilbao Guggenheim Museum (1994–97), any thing can be any shape. Gehry has restored expression to a central place.

To seek the tragic in modern architecture, we may have to follow Adolf Loos' injunction to return to the tomb and the monument, where physical functionality, as such, has no weight. In Carlo Scarpa's tomb and cemetery for the Brion-Vega family at San Vito (1970–72), however, it is not the purpose of the building that affects us so much as the extreme concentration on detail. If anyone were to convince us that 'God is in the detail' it would be Scarpa. It is difficult to explain this effect. We are somehow dislocated from our ordinary view of things; we are not returned to the object-in-itself, however, but to a sense of the importance of seeing, an opening of the inner eye.

James Stirling is very different; he is brusque where Scarpa is precious, but there is an extraordinary moment at the Staatsgalerie, Stuttgart, where the main gallery, with its covered cornice, draws back to admit the bulge of the central drum, creating an enormous compression of space that, again, refreshes our

sense of being alive. Both Scarpa and Stirling are architects who question the ordinary and expose us to the unexpected, and renew our sense of the human condition.

With Tadao Ando's well-known Church of the Light (Osaka, 1987–9), we have a strange reversal of values. The Christian cross was always seen in the West as solid, the indubitable *thing* on which the god-hero was killed. Ando, from outside the Christian fold, is able to see it as an opening, and therefore as space, undeniably renewing our sense of its symbolic meaning. This drawing back from the oppression of Western muscularity can also produce a Zen sense of the fullness of space, through underlining the potency of emptiness, as we saw in his 'O' House of 1998.

These are examples of an architecture that is not directed squarely at the idea of mechanism, but that still works through the physical to engender a sense of values that I would roughly describe as spiritual. Does this approach the tragic? No, but it allows the possibility of the tragic to come close so that it can be precipitated in the observer, who is saturated with an emotion. Architecture can be expressive, and the tragic is not precluded by any principle that I know of.

Certain architects have seen themselves as tragic figures, and Charles Jencks has shown how that category applies to Le Corbusier. A reader of Nietzsche, Le Corbusier saw himself as a protagonist of great art, engaged in a struggle to balance the intellectual and the lyrical in order to realise the potential of the epoch.

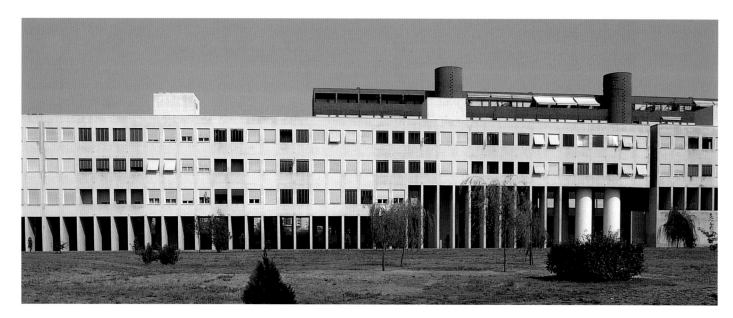

The fat columns are not rational; they deliberately cancel out the rational premise of the entire design.

Above
Aldo Rossi, Gallaratese
Housing, Milan, (1970–3).

Something of this struggle adheres to many of his works: if they are not the staging of tragedy they undeniably have tragic force. The buildings at Chandigarh, like Louis Kahn's Sher-e-Bangla Nagara Dakar, Bangladesh (1962–87), address human life in heroic terms, and raise an awareness of the power of hubris, the fatal flaw that brings the hero down.

But my choice of the tragic in architecture comes to rest on the image of Aldo Rossi's Gallaratese Housing in Milan. It is itself a comment on Chandigarh, I have no doubt, and just as Corbu mixes the machine with the grandiloquent, so does Rossi. Throughout its length the building is supported by concrete columns arranged on a rational module, as in the heroic buildings of early modernism. But at one point the rhythm is broken by two 'fat' columns that introduce a false note.

The fat columns are not rational; they deliberately cancel out the rational premise of the entire design. The break in the regularity creates a framing device, proclaiming an ironic self-awareness. It thereby induces a matching awareness in us, placing us in the role of audience confronting something deliberately staged. Rossi made many drawings of this motif – clearly it was intentionally a figure, in the way that Scully applies this term to Rothko. In its combination of the lyrical and the intellectual, it speaks for the impossibility of achieving perfection.

In that sense, and for those who can read the book of architecture, it makes a truly tragic statement. But this value is only apparent when the built work is interpreted in context.

If we consider how important context is for the staging of opera, we can begin to see how architecture, once built, takes on *as setting* a fullness that it does not have within its own autonomy. Bernard Tschumi appreciated this long ago in his *Manhattan Transcripts*.[3] In opera, we observe how music, libretto, lighting, choreography, staging, casting even – all independent areas of decision, all separate systems – are separately nebulous, but when coordinated, they can achieve a dramatic effect and move the spirit in powerful ways. At the moment when a busy stage empties, lights reduce to a single spot focused centre stage on a man and women, and the orchestra goes from full spate to solo oboe, we have no difficulty in construing the meaning. The performance takes the initiative. Architecture, too, can enter into performance, profiting from our desire to see life transmuted into art. As the setting of social space, in its wide reach from the quotidian to the moment of personal epiphany, it *is* capable of responding to emotion, and of placing the entirely personal into the entirely social. ⏃

The text was adapted by the author for publication from his presentation given at the Royal Academy Forum, 'The Tragic in Art and Architecture', in London on 16 March 2000.

Notes
1. In my original presentation I was making particular reference to the theme of Minimalism because it had been the subject of the previous Royal Academy forum on 8 December 1998. See 'Aspects of Minimal Architecture' II, *Architectural Design*, vol 69, no 5/6, May–June 1999, pp 8–17.
2. Sean Scully, 'Against the dying of his own light: mystery and sadness in Rothko's work', *Times Literary Supplement*, 6 November 1998.
3. Bernard Tschumi, *Manhattan Transcripts*, Academy Editions (London), 1981.

The Disorder of Order,

Behind the 'meaningless arithmetical mantra' of the grid, argues John Outram, is the forbidden cave of riches that is history, sealed up by the tragedy of modernism with a powerful taboo. To open and explore it, he suggests, would be to discover the fleshed out, still-breathing body of architecture, of which the grid is only the cryptic treasure map.

and After

The Act of Foundation –
One of the Four Kinds
of Time. (After Paul Ricoeur.)

John Outram

'Nothing'
Drawing made for a lecture to the
architects of Houston in 1996.
In the Beginning there was Nothing.
Paul Ricoeur tells us, in *Time and
Narrative*, Book One (1983), that St
Augustine argued that God, before
He created, created nothing.

'Nothing and its Double'
Drawing made for a lecture to the
architects of Houston in 1996.
Everything that comes into being
comes into existence in the
company of its opposite, its other,
its double. Black comes with white,
life with death and ham with
melon. Why should nothing be the
exception? So what is the negation
of nothing? Surely it is not
something: nothings eat
somethings for breakfast. No, the
only thing strong enough to oppose
nothing is another negation. So
when negation brought nothing into
being (or was it the other way
round?) they began to circle around
each other, aware that they had a
problem. Two nothings were going
to be difficult neighbours.

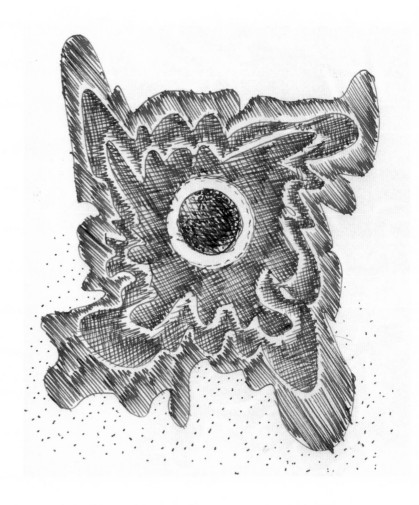

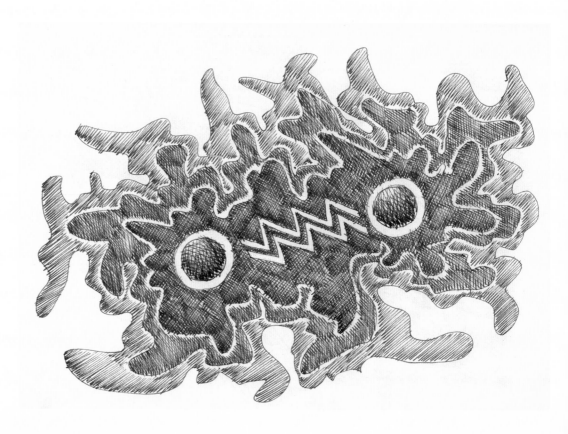

'The first thing I do', remarked Mies van der Rohe, 'is to divine the grid', which varies, he went on to indicate, according to site and programme. When I met Mies in 1959 someone asked him why he didn't paint his steel white, so as to make it light. Mies replied that steel was heavy. He never spoke at length.

The black steel grids of Mies were all that was left after the stony ore of the antique was crushed and burnt in the holocaust of the 20th century. Mies poured the heavy, formless, flow of metal to sink, like a branding iron, into the soft green grass of Illinois. What form could this inert plasticity take except that of the irreducible residue, like a shadow left by an atomic fireball, of the Neoclassical architectural practice that Mies both knew and rejected? What remained, trenched into the earth, cast into the sky like black ink lines from his rough watercolour paper, but the puerile computations of the canonic orders? It seems that when all else failed, a meaningless arithmetical mantra could remain, to serve as a mute memorial. Mies' cindered skeletons, as eternally durable as the monomolecular filaments of carbon left after the fabric is burnt away, remain etched in the sky of America to remind her of all that was lost, at some point, on the journey to the Promised Land.

It was in that sort of place, standing on an old iron bridge over the Riviere Rouge in Winnipeg, that I decided to become an architect. The bridge trembled under mid 20th-century traffic. The river was desolate with industrial ruin and pollution. What was its redness? The blood of nature? A speedboat cut across its welling muscles, laying them open. I imagined the river as a street from the India of my upbringing, thronged with white-robed people, externally animate, internally still. The derelict banks rose up like the tiers of a theatre whose buildings formed a city in my mind.

On the one side was St Boniface, the French-Canadian quarter, where people lived in stone apartment houses and put chairs in the street to watch television through the shop windows. On the other side the old, sociable 'porch' houses were being rebuilt as 'ranch' houses. Their roofs hit the ground, their vision turned inwards, the thermostat registered winter and the imitation fire blazed in the random-rubble hearth. The house became a plywood satellite marooned in ballistic space. A vegetable storm of disenfranchised shrubberies heaved and waved where once a calm sea of grass lazily lapped wooden porticoes. The colonists, once

so sure of their anchorage, were now to be dispersed again, each flying before the winds of change, hopping wavelengths in videospace, unsure what flag of fashion they should fly.

What are Frank Gehry's buildings but the ballooning internal spirit of the ranch house, inflamed by the silvery palettes of cyberspace, floating free of any civic moorings. His 'fish scales' are roof shingles. They hit the ground like a virgin's veil, hiding the body of an architecture that is lost in space.

The period of the unitary 'melting pot' culture of Americanisation was over. North America, newly equipped with automobiles, television and air conditioning, was about to fissure, regressing into pre-American ethnicities. In the centre of Winnipeg the coal-stove-heated trams had not long to run. Every other fine 19th- and early 20th-century masonry building was being demolished to make way for the tatty car-parking sites that were the main landscape innovation introduced by the great life space churn whose tax revenues would ultimately bring America her victory in the Cold War, and leave her cities in ruins.

Even so, Mies was right: the first rite of architecture is the 'bringing of the Fire', the Promethean revolt against nature. This is why architecture is *persona non grata* today. The cult of sustainability, like all such, has its taboos. One of them, it is very clear, is the quality of humanity itself. Yet it is human beings who sustain cultures, not nature. We have to *want* to sustain the onerous complexity of civilisation. A green civilisation will be no different. It will depend upon the will, energy, intelligence and enthusiasm of man, not nature. Nothing is so sustainable as the abandoned ruin of a once-great and beautiful city.

The Maya, tired of their dizzying cultural superstructure, walked away from it back into the jungle, where they stayed for 200 years before being brought out again by the Aztecs, perhaps the most terrifyingly coercive culture known to man. The defect of the Maya was purely technical: their infrastructure was pathetic. The Aztecs did not rectify it. They just added more terror. It is important that things be 'made to work' for ordinary people in the most ordinary way. It is one of the virtues of the American ethic.

When Mies invoked his grid, he called down upon his unsuspecting site the disorder of order. As in the killing and eating of animals, we feel guilt when we build. The expiation of Mies was to render his buildings invisible – made of glass. What can one call this but a cheap trick, hardly worthy of a snake-oil salesman? Le Corbusier seems even more disturbed. He ordered that the new cities should be built (roads and all) up in the air on stilts so that the 'rolling fields and rushing rivers' of the primordial site should be preserved. Were these early 20th-century architects cases for the shrink, or what?

Yet the 20th century believed them and faithfully

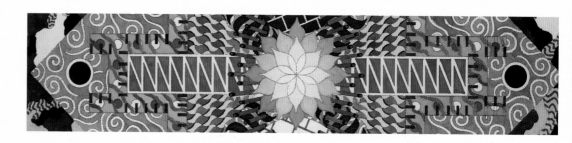

'The Novelty'
A fragment of the JOA design for the Shaper Ceiling, Duncan Hall, Rice University, Houston, USA. JOA, 1992–7. The origin of the universe has been described as being due to a 'wobble'. Perhaps it was a wobble in the life of nothing caused by the sight of its opposite: another nothing. By this argument creation was an accident that was bound to happen. God blinked. When He opened His eyes was it the same nothing that he saw, or its negation? Creation was the product of the instability of nothing. It was caused by nothing and, well, is it for nothing? Beginning with a bang, it will end, for humanity at least, with another bang–a piece of stellar debris or some lava-boil erupting from our sluggish core will wipe us out. Until then we can, at least, remain clear-headed.

'Shadow'
A fragment of the JOA design for the Shaper Ceiling, Duncan Hall, Rice University, Houston, USA. JOA, 1992–7. The 20th century was the only century when humanity was unable to build itself a life space in which it could represent its understanding of the larger picture. Phenomenology leads to sex, drugs and rock-and-roll. It is not enough to found philosophy and it has been the death of architecture. There can be no 'vision' without that point in infinity at which the parallel rays thrown out by every eye meet. Today we have that black hole in working order. We know the direction in which that terminus which consumes even the most decentred discourse of a Francophone Fountain of Différance. We have a big bang back in some sort of working order and can do an architectural microcosmos again. So why is the bang eight-lobed and yellow? Well, it's not a photograph and its about us rather than the quark family. So make what you like of it.

The bang was a 'pure event', a synaptic frenzy, the first protest demo in the binocular vision of pure blindness. It was not light, or energy, or power. But it held the blueprints of them all inside its gambler's dice. Fire is its mundane embodiment today. Every fire that burns on earth shooting its interstellar dust, like spit that misses the spittoon, into our clear atmosphere, rehearses the 'act of foundation'. Out of it came Light. But light is proven only by its 'shadow': darkness. Colour is the stain that matter leaves on light, all the way down to its death in the fagged-out freezer of 'space'. A planet of matter circles the sun of fire. On one side it is white, on the other black. But, as Professor Keith Cooper of Rice advised, 'only an architect denotes a planet as solid by building it of cinderblock'.

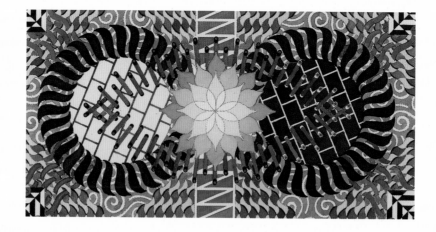

followed their prescription. The crime of culture was absolved and the carpet of concrete unrolled. Le Corbusier's peculiar achievement was to ensure that the main pay-off to the 'crime of construction' – a comfortable, inhabitable city, with wide pavements, arcades and sheltered streets – remained unachievable. Corbu gave us undercroft parking lots and hurricane-force down draughts.

Mies made air conditioning absolutely necessary. He thereby polluted the air of the tropics, the beautiful, soft, warm, moist, aromatic air of the gardens of Edinnu, with the hammering of compressors. I call this the bird song of Houston. He also made every city building look inwards upon itself because nothing but mirror glass reflecting other mirror

his ruins and get up every morning and look at the monstrous disaster of his golden age from on high, behind plate-glass walls like searchlights that would inflame, cast in images as clear as the sun itself, a natural order worthy of Mankind. Beatriz Colomina has shown how, shorn of the transcendent illusions of perspective, the Western gaze turned outwards from the shadows on the philosopher's cave to ignite a holocaust consuming everything that was not perfect.[1] This cleansing of the augean stables applied especially to man and his works.

But what then? Having begun, the architects of the 20th century seemed unable to continue. They remained frozen by the sublime terror of the first and final act. Infinity was inscribed but, after this, the fire of Prometheus cooled in their hands.

Their play could not progress because the script was

There is no uglier scene today than the view from some high twentieth-century building. One sees nothing but ant-hills filled with people – each occupying a tiny room. Nothing of grandeur or scale is visible.

glass remained in view outside. There is no uglier scene today than the view from some high 20th-century building. One sees nothing but ant hills filled with people – each occupying a tiny room. Nothing of grandeur or scale is visible. Such a piling up of smallness with no translation, no pay-off, no 'leap' into bigness, is pathetic. The late 20th-century 'boardroom view' surveys the biggest failure in planned urbanity, ever.

So what went wrong? What is this 21st-century city but grid upon grid ad infinitum? But that is the point. It is frozen into a block of black, Miesian, ice, like a brain preserved for the moment, for which a 'technology' will unlock the means to revive once-active synapses. For the disorder of order begins at the beginning, with the invocation of that moment, infinitely deferred, when all things were equal and no time existed except the eternal present of an infinite repetition – trees passing in an endless forest that has no edge. Mies, reading Aquinas, knew that this 'time before time' had to be invoked, embodied and, like an epiphany of the negation that must always accompany creation, be made real.

Le Corbusier wanted to destroy every building constructed by man and plant huge forests over

taboo. The elaborate architectural sequences were all locked behind a door called 'the past'. Without these forbidden charts, hidden under thick layers of dust, it proved impossible to navigate the monstrous horizons that must be breached by the Flow of Time if Fate is to be married to Will and Infinitude to return as Personality. Those qualified to enter found themselves in Ali Baba's cave. Everything was alluring. One could stay as long as one liked. Historians stayed forever. But if and when one left, one passed through a small room where all memory of the cave's contents was erased. Out in the sunlit world of the future, one remembered nothing of the past. The reason for this was that it had been decided that nothing 'worked' in the future that had worked in the past. This decision was irrevocable and was itself, like the past, under lock and key.

Certain explorers, some authorised, some not, hearing of this forbidden treasure, obtained access to it. They bypassed the machines that erased memory and began to loot the cave. The past entered into general circulation, but in an illegal, unauthorised, exciting, way as something bad, something forbidden. It was considered chic to mix the past with the future, playing elusive intellectual games with its dusty, cobwebbed images. Bordellos and casinos manufactured whole forbidden worlds called Egypt and Paris and even New York. But, under and over it all, the big taboo still held.

'Raft of the Founders'
Part of the ceiling of one of the
Palazzi Massimi, Campo Marzo,
Rome, when it was being restored
by the team who had just finished
restoring the Sistine Chapel.
1992–3.

The architectural medium requires
that the ceiling of a room is an
'entablature'. The entablature in
most cultures, occidental as well as
oriental, shows on the interior, as a
'coffer', *coffre* (French), or *cassone*
(Italian): a chest of valuables.
The privileged occupant of the
interior had a view up into this chest
as its *caelum* (Latin sky) had been
chiselled away by a *coelum* (Latin
chisel). What is it that this peculiar
cavity reveals? Is it a contrarotating
sunflower, burnished in gold and
clearly the precursor to the Convair
XFY1, Pogo and other vertical-lift-
off machines?

'The Ark as Cargo of the Raft'
A coffer from the ceiling above.
The grammatical meaning of the
coffre is as the roof of one of the
doorless cavitations of the
primordial vacancies in brute
matter described by Serlio as
'rooms'. Larger rooms are
measured by the number of these
'standard hypostylar modules' that
are revealed above them. The lexical
meaning is more accessible. Yet
because lexicons always link beyond
the medium, these revelations are
more 'fantastic'. Here the *cassone*
contains the valuables carried on
the Entabled Trabica during its
voyage as raft of the founders. The
primary cargo, denoted by the
golden floret, is the lens of a
pinhole camera in the large cavity
above the floret. So far as one can
tell, from the infinite repetition of
these small glowing 'points', the
cargo above is always the hearth
fire, ancestral ash cone of civic
sacrifices, light in the darkness of
ignorance and sun in the blackness
of entropic history.

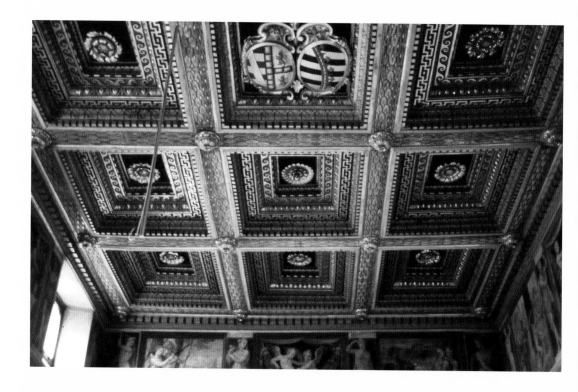

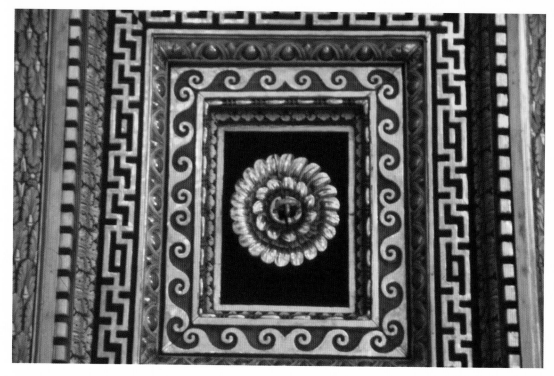

The past was not really serious. It played no role in the future.

This is because everyone still agreed that the past was 'unusable'. But what if it were not? What if someone invented a way of making it work? What if someone built a huge core-drill that could ream out the centres of the giant stone columns of temples and make them into crawlways and ductways, filling them with machines and pipes and wires? What if someone invented a way of tunnelling secretly throughout the huge carved entablatures that rested on the columns. so that these hitherto inanimate and useless quarries of stone were filled with the electromechanical viscera of giant robots? Seen with X-ray eyes as cubic lattices of service ducts and scaffoldings for maintenance engineers, and light pipes, and gondolas, and sun blinds and other environmental aids, would not the giant, and hitherto useless, structures of antiquity begin to be conceivable as useful to our own, 'modern', future?

What if someone invented a way of tunnelling secretly throughout the huge carved entablatures that rested on the columns so that these hitherto inanimate and useless quarries of stone were filled with the electromechanical viscera of giant robots?

And what if someone invented a way of getting the structures that used these lattices and scaffoldings and claddings to 'build themselves', in such a way that, like the skeleton, viscera, nerves and skin of the mammalian genera, nothing was required to bring them into being except their own bodies?

What if someone invented a giant stone column of a peculiar form such that one could walk through it and drive automobiles through it. Such a column would no longer block the passage of people and vehicles like the dumb, rocky monoliths of the Egyptians or the Greeks. It would, on the contrary, facilitate, ease and encourage *commoditas*, the central utility of the Vitruvian triad. Would not such an overwhelmingly – and even childishly – simple equipment of service columns and circulation columns allow one to entertain the thought that

the rational felicities of beaux-arts planning, instead of being the footprints of a Greco-Gothic spider high on steroids, were now (as they never were in the 19th century) the most functional way to plan large sites and buildings?

Then what if someone invented a way of inscribing 'glyphs' (figures and colours) that 'wrote' on the ample surfaces of these 'antique' members, and the even ampler picture planes (huge floors and ceilings) that they enframed, in such a way that this picture-writing made sense to people today, instead of just to art historians and casino operators. What if such a form of pictorial writing based its technique upon the everyday usages of post-perspectival supermarket graphics (with their brilliant formalities and information-rich iconics), and the received ideas of contemporary philosophy and science? What if such a technique created a raiment for architecture that, like the new skin of a snake, was brilliant and fresh. Would this new, modern, decor not be more 'antique', (because more 'original' – like the real, coloured-all-over, waxed and shiny Parthenon) than the even bleached stones of 15th-century antiquity?

Would that not be a prescription for a modern version of the architectural microcosm? Would that not enable a group of people to share a vision of the cosmos revealed as they conceive it actually to be: as reality rather than appearance, conception rather than perception, vision rather than view? Would not this restore the central kernel of the architectural technique of the past as a contemporary, practical tool?

What if these techniques combined into a method that proved capable of deliberately foreplanned futuristic 'environmental engineering' in all three of the Vitruvian categories of the mechanical, the social and the conceptual life space. Would not then the past begin to appear, just *begin* to appear (like a dreadful apparition threatening to overturn all the received ideologies of 20th-century architectural practice), not entirely useless and dysfunctional, as was always assumed throughout the last century? Might not then the seals be broken upon this doggedly misunderstood treasure house. Might not it be time to bring its contents out into the laboratory of the present and examine it in the light of the idea that there are things which, like the obscure moulds of the rainforest, really 'work' when they are decoded, deciphered and encrypted?

Until the 20th century, men did architecture like sleepwalkers. In the 20th century they decided to wake up and leave architecture in the land of dreams. The 20th century ended with the human life space as a man-made nightmare. Can we keep awake in the 21st century and do architecture as well? ☐

Notes
1. Beatriz Colomina, *Privacy and Publicity*, MIT Press (Cambridge, Mass), 1994.

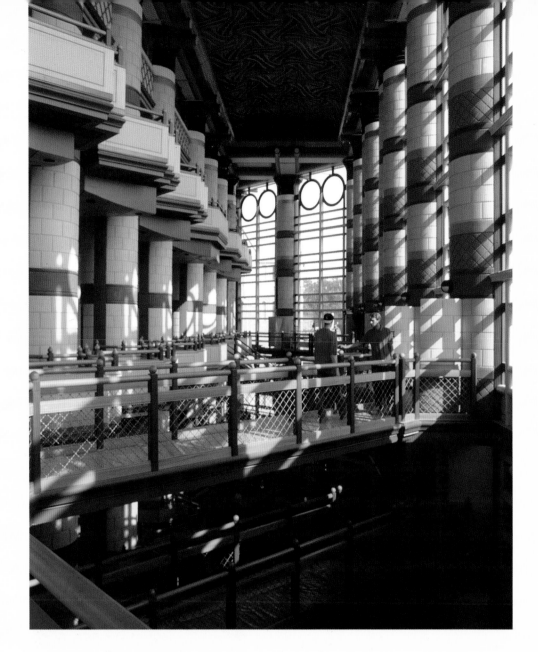

'Travelling Light'
A view of the Gallery, the Space of Appearances, of the Judge Institute of Management Studies, Cambridge University, England. JOA, 1991-5.

Should the occupant of such an architectural, 'trabeated' interior wish a better view of the *cassone* interior he must strip away the enrafting structure that veils the view up into the caelum-ceiling. He will then be able to enumerate and describe the contents of the Ark itself. This is an invitation either to the inscription of an empty vessel, voyaging without the proper cargo with which it will sustain and plant the new foundation, such as the one we had no alternative but to record in the ceiling of the Judge Institute; or it is an invitation to the pleasant task of cataloguing the plenitude of colonising tools that we were able to record in the vault (that is to say, the securely 'enrafted' container) of Duncan Hall.

'The Fully-Loaded Ark'
The 55 x 70 foot shaper ceiling erected in its vault.

The enrafted cargo enclosed in the *cassone* of the Faculty of Computation, Rice University, has already been shown to descend from nothing to the existence of matter, light and the serpentine oceans. The taxonomy continues with the elaboration of two canonic histories of the 'time of foundation': an oriental and an occidental history.

A technical point: This ceiling was designed and drawn, by John Outram, as an A1 watercolour. It was then photographed, in the City of London, on to a 10 x 8 inch transparency and rotary drum scanned into a 780Mb file. This was then 'tiled' electronically, via Live Picture and DeBableser, by Anthony Charnley, of JOA, into 234 2 x 8 foot strips. No colours were changed at this stage. The strips were printed, from one 650 Mb CD, supplied by JOA to Scanachrome Ltd of Skelmersdale, on to a fire-resistant and acoustically transparent 'canvas' sourced from Ohio. Colour balancing was done, by Outram, on Scanachrome's digitally controlled four-colour acrylic paint spray-paint machines. The fabrics were sent to Decoustic Ltd of Toronto and wrapped around 1 inch-thick fibreglass ceiling tiles. The tiles were erected in a curved hidden-fixing metal grid, in 48 hours. The commission was given by Rice Board to JOA on 12 December 1995. The ceiling was erected by the end of August 1996. The cost was one tenth that of the *'buon fresco'* ceiling that JOA failed to install in the Judge Institute. Being 'modern' in its entire technology, and produced by architects, without any intervention by 'artists', it is vastly to be preferred and adds to the Judge ceiling an entirely new dimension to the ability of our profession to intellectually script the critical surfaces of our buildings. Because the pigment is in paint and not ink, it is light fast. One day we may hope for sufficient progress to have been made in iconic engineering to enable the 'inscriptions' of a building to be changed to accord with changed ideas.

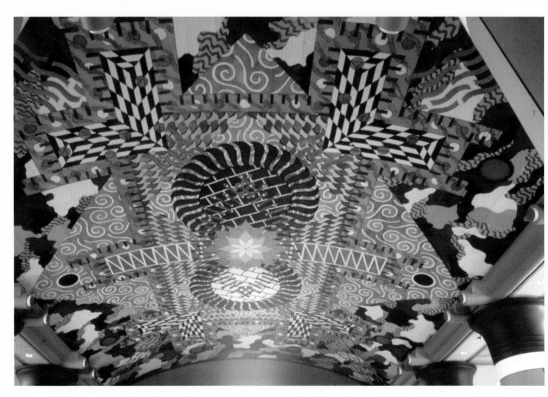

'The Eastern Story'
A drawing by John Outram made to illustrate
the metaphorical 'event-horizons' of the
Oriental Flood and Ark Myth.
In the oriental version the rootless raft,
wandering in search of its 'fruitful
grounding' is transfixed by an act of will, a
re-enactment of the big bang, which anchors
it to the 'submarine mountain'. This watery
tumescence, guarded by the serpent Vrta,
representative of inertia, infinity and the
endless return of the same upon itself, is
sundered and split into four quarters. The
dark sun, the 'fire in the rock', is released
and rises up a predetermined progression,
emerging from the waters, floating on them
as an earthy lotus, breathing forth to the
four quarters on the airy medium of the
voice and finally achieving the fiery eye of
the cakra. Only the fifth frame is missing
from this film: that of 'thought', represented
on the columns of the Martell Hall by the
smooth, curving, black capitals, devoid of all
iconic specificity except that of an ultimate,
reflective darkness.

The grounding of the ark of the founders
goes unrecorded. The ramshackle vehicle of
their voyage, the green boat of reeds, albeit
each filled with 'trabeated' fire, is
shipwrecked and sundered. But the violence
of the founding act ensures that the cycle of
creation pursues its predetermined path
with a force and brilliance, all the way up to
its final apotheosis and subsequent collapse,
ready for the next cataclysmic regeneration.

'The Western Story'
The Shaper Ceiling over the Martell Hall, in
Duncan Hall, the Faculty of Computational
Engineering for Rice University, Houston,
Texas.
In this other history the raft is imperishable
reason. Its Cartesian span, infinite as any
reticulation, enmeshes the planet, rendered
here as a blue square of ocean – square
because the earth is solid, blue because it
belongs, mainly, to the whales. The time of
the Occident is the linear time of progress,
not the cyclic time of the Orient. Progress
cannot collapse and begin again, springing
afresh from the ruins of the old dynasty. It
has to press forever onwards, becoming one
with time itself. The sun and moon cycle
across the sands and rivers of the yellow
'sand bars' of the Western ark whose
'canonic beams' are cored with the blood
of power.

This wandering craft, far from
shattering to be reconstituted out of the
debris of the expected periodic cataclysm,
comes to carry the entire history of the
earth. Entry to its palace is under six
gateways, altars whose horned acroteria are
the leaves of the new crop which the
voyagers carry to the new foundation. Even
the four shattered quarters of the primordial
tumulus that once buried the 'germ that
was always there', obscured by the coil of
time, are caught in its reticulated embrace.
All that escapes from the 'embrace of
reason' are the four 'outspeakings' that flow
from the centre of combustion, like roads
stretching out into the void of the cosmos.
These 'heavenly' blue waves expel their
ethereal refreshment into an unformed
field of light and darkness, fire and energy.
Is anyone listening?

Tragedy is the echo which returns when
the distance between what ought to be, and
what is, can be measured by the
outstretched rule of a canonic law. How can
any history measure up to the rule of the
tragic until it can know what it is to be:
'as things should be'?

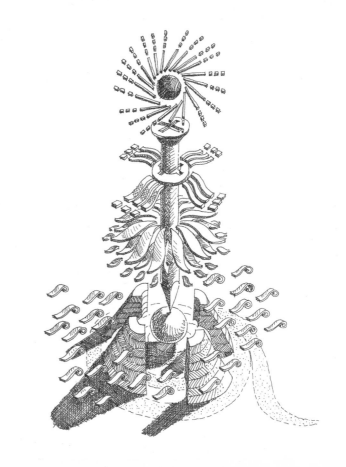

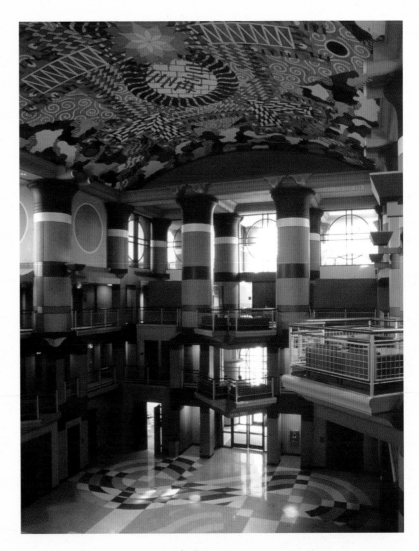

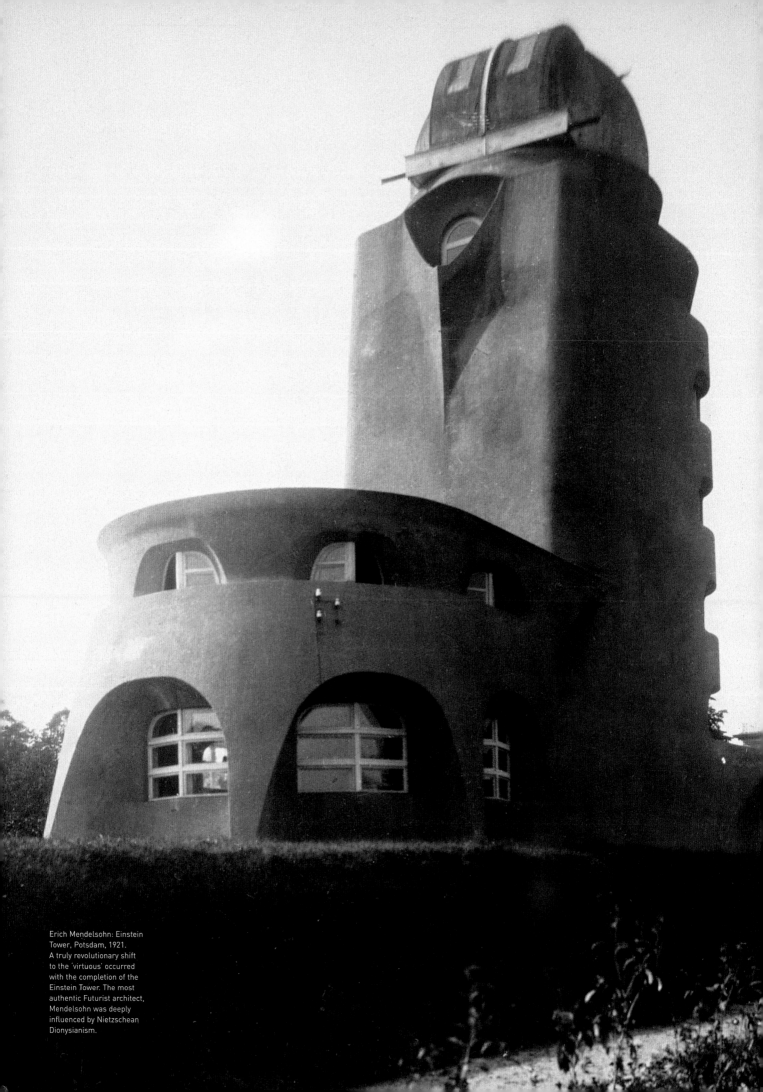

Erich Mendelsohn: Einstein
Tower, Potsdam, 1921.
A truly revolutionary shift
to the 'virtuous' occurred
with the completion of the
Einstein Tower. The most
authentic Futurist architect,
Mendelsohn was deeply
influenced by Nietzschean
Dionysianism.

The Virtuous Tower

In the late medieval period certain classical ideas were dramatically transformed in ways that significantly reconfigured traditional semantic networks. This is particularly evident in the Hermetic writings, where concepts such as 'wholeness' and 'virtue' – qualities associated with Aristotelian tragedy – acquired mystical, supernatural, even erotic meanings. In this article, David Hamilton Eddy explores the sensuous implications of the use of such concepts following their migration to architecture.

FR Leavis was determined that theory and ideology should never distract us from the spontaneous, lively experience of literature and culture. His dictum, *mutatis mutandis*, provides us with a clear means to the evaluation of architecture.

In the late medieval period, *c*1450, 'integrity' signified a sense of soundness, wholeness and completeness.[2] This Aristotelian concept was important in Hermetic discourse, along with that of 'virtue', or 'superiority or excellence; unusual ability, merit or distinction ... physical strength, force or energy'.[3] To the late medieval mind, the 'virtuous' was 'endowed with or possessed of inherent or natural virtue or power (often of a magical, occult or supernatural kind); (making it) potent in effect, influence or operation'.[4] It is in this sense of effective power that the adjective 'virtuous' is appropriate to architecture.

In European history, the tower or spire is not a classical but a late medieval and gothic form, and in its scholastic context, the Aristotelian/ Hermetic idea of virtue would apply. The Gothic architecture of soaring stone and forbidding gargoyle is absolutely 'virtuous' in the powerful, magical, occult and indeed, supernatural, sense. The Gothic cathedral was not just to do with life in the Leavisian sense: it more or less defined life and embodied it spiritually and psychologically, and it was precisely this powerful effect that Romanticism attempted to resurrect.

The property of virtue in buildings is intrinsic to their sensuous effect, constituted in that plasticity of form and surface that has been largely abandoned in the 20th century. Seeking after virtue and the virtuous in building cannot extend to iconic skyscrapers, particularly as promulgated under the aegis of the International Style and the mannered control epitomised by Mies van der Rohe's Seagram building (1956–9) inasmuch as the box-like structure of these buildings, with or without decoration, denies us the virtuous qualities we are seeking. In a larger sense, the problem with the boxy structure is that it is primarily rationalistic, geometric and abstract. It is Apollonian rather than Dionysian. It bears no relationship to anything found in the natural world, unlike classical and Gothic architectures which refer to trees, forests and so on. Even crystals are rarely square. Yet, we have been so conditioned to the experience of rectilinearity in architecture that to reject such significant buildings as 'unvirtuous' seems eccentric if not perverse.

But the invocation of the Aristotelian tragic demand of a complete 'action' represented through compositional integrity, requires us also to focus on the special meaning of virtue in European history, for it is in this that architectural and musical experience has its prerational grip. The fact is that Dionysus takes precedence over Apollo. As Freud pointed out, rationality developed in order to gain a degree of fearful control over the tyrannical demands of pleasure.[5] Virtue in the sense used here seeks to celebrate and extend pleasure, to rescue it from the equally tyrannical demands of the superego, not to deny it by obsessing on rational rectilinearity. In other words, do we experience the sense of wholeness, of magic, of occult power, in short of life with all its richness, subtlety, beauty and horror, in a boxy structure, however sublime or large – or do we in fact, experience the opposite of life, the opposite of desire and of hope?

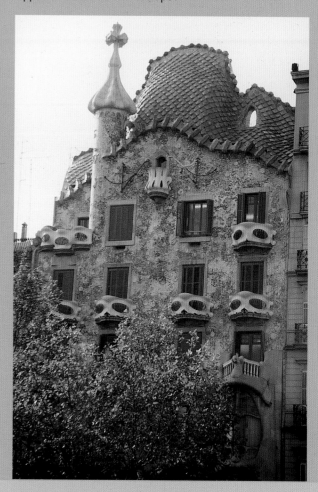

Antonio Gaudí is a modern exception, in that his work, based as it is on forms derived from the curves of catenary chains, extends the Gothic. That is, his outrageous, emotional and inflammatory forms have been developed from the force of gravity, in the way of the Gothic, much as the boughs of a tree are conditioned by way of gravity. His architecture is a literally wonderful expression of Gothic virtue – reminding us of the beauty and complexity of natural forms – the last authentic Gothic buildings of Europe. In this sense, Gaudí's work is both shocking and deeply traditional, even conservative, in that it is imbued with visual narrative in Catalan legend and myth. The roof of the Casa Battló (1904–6), as Charles Jencks has pointed out, represents the corpse of the Spanish dragon killed by St George, patron saint of Barcelona.[6] The image was always an integral part of the Gothic experience in the Middle Ages.

To experience sensuous and, with Gaudí, even sensual, architecture is to experience life in the virtuous, Leavisian manner. One cannot enter a Gaudí building without one's senses being heightened and aroused, one's body made sympathetic to the dignified eroticism around it.

One cannot enter a Gaudí building without one's senses being heightened and aroused, one's body made sympathetic to the dignified eroticism around it.

Not for nothing did Michelangelo Antonioni arrange for the lovers (Jack Nicholson and Maria Schneider) in The Passenger (1975) to meet within a Gaudí building. But the truly revolutionary shift to the virtuous occurred not with the Sagrada Familia in Barcelona in 1903, but in 1921 with the completion of the Einstein Tower in Potsdam by Erich Mendelsohn.

Influenced by the Futurist architects Antonio Sant'Elia and Mario Chiattone, and especially by the Futurist sculptor Umberto Boccioni, Mendelsohn was in fact the only authentic and successful Futurist architect.[7] This was partly to do with his ability to translate what for the Italians was never realised into built form. But there were other reasons, at the heart of Futurism itself. There had been a degree of opportunism, for example, in Filippo Marinetti's adoption of Nuove Tendenze, the group of Sant'Elia and Chiattone, into mainstream Futurism in 1914. Marinetti needed Sant'Elia et al to envisage the new Futurist city, but Carlo

Carrà, for example, came to doubt their Futurist credentials.[8] Thus, it was Mendelsohn, influenced by Boccioni , who developed a more integrated and dynamic architecture which can be properly called 'Futurist'. The development of electrically welded steel reinforcement allowed Mendelsohn to defy gravity in his later, cantilevered, 'floating' buildings. This use of reinforced concrete also permitted a dynamic plasticity. That in the Einstein Tower facilitated the expression of a furious, blatant eroticism, anticipating the streamlined, fleshy curves of American industrial design of the 1930s.[9]

The Einstein Tower signals a real shift in sensibility. Its Dionysian phallic shape, its curved, streamlined, near-symmetrical form, embodies animal not vegetable virtue, and implies the primacy of sexual desire. (In a 1923 lecture, Mendelsohn refers to admiring 'the muscle play of the naked body'.)[10] The Einstein Tower represents not just the 20th century's fascination with sexuality, but a Nietzschean, post-Judeo-Christian reversion to paganism within the heart of technology. The Futurists were iconoclastic anarchists who saluted the prostitute as well as the machine. Marinetti attacked what he saw as the sentimental and false nature of relations between men and women as represented by l'amore. Similarly, the Futurist feminist Valentine de Saint-Point argued that men and women were equal in their capacity for lust or desire, which she defined as a powerful and natural source of dynamic energy that could lead to the liberation of the spirit. Italo Tavolato developed these themes in the Futurist magazine Lacerba in a satirical celebration of prostitution.[11] Mendelsohn, for his part, was deeply influenced by Nietzschean Dionysianism – he made continual references to Dionysian energies, alluded at least once to Zarathustra in his letters and gave a lecture on Nietzsche in Munich at the salon of one Baroness von Bissing. It can be said of Mendelsohn's work that it anticipates the peculiar modern duality of our fascination with technology and pornography.

The technology of the Einstein Tower, for example, is contained within the streamlined surface of the building, just as the Merlin engine is contained within the streamlined surface of the Spitfire, or the XK engine within the Jaguar XK120. The Einstein Tower is similarly a functioning device, a solar observatory with its mirrors and lenses supported by a rectilinear wooden and steel structure on a heavy concrete base.[12] Even the streamlining of the surface has a functional purpose: it helps to obviate vibration from high winds, which would have disturbed and distorted the microscopic readings taken in the underground laboratory. Here then, we might say that Apollo and Dionysus have worked in harmony.

It becomes clear that we are confronting a new/old definition of virtue; one that connects with medieval

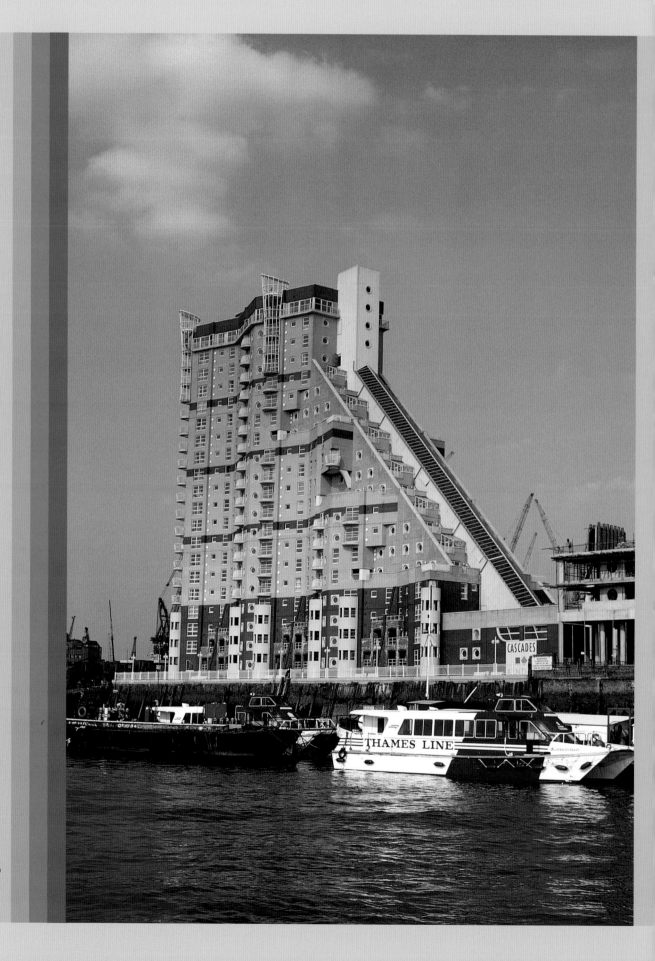

CZWG: Cascades, Isle of Dogs, London, 1988. This virtuous housing block embodies the search for armistice between the intellect and the senses that lies at the heart of tragedy.

Notes
1. FR Leavis quoted in Ian MacKillop, *FR Leavis: A Life in Criticism*, Allen Lane (London) 1995.
2. David Hamilton Eddy 'Unwilling the Freedom Spirit', *The Times Higher Education Supplement*, 17 June 1990.
3. *Oxford English Dictionary*.
4. Ibid.
5. Sigmund Freud, *The Ego and the Id*, Hogarth Press (London), 1927.
6. Charles Jencks *The Language of Post-Modern Architecture*, Academy Editions (London), 1977.
7. Katherine James, in 'Erich Mendelsohn and the Architecture of German Modernism', confirms my earlier work 'Erich Mendelsohn: the Secret Futurist', *The Times Higher Education Supplement*, 24 August 1990, in asserting the influence of Boccioni's sculpture on the Einstein Tower. She cites a hitherto unknown letter from Mendelsohn to his wife (31 October 1912), in which he expresses his interest in Futurist art.
8. See Caroline Tisdall and Angelo Bozzolla, *Futurism*, Oxford University Press (New York and Toronto), 1978, p 125, and my own unpublished monograph on Futurism, 'Mendelsohn and streamlining: The Birth of the Future'.
9. Nikolaus Pevsner, too, referred to Sant'Elia's influence on Mendelsohn, connecting it as well with the idea of the streamlined in *Outline of European Architecture*, Penguin Books (London), 1960.
10. Erich Mendelsohn 'The International Consensus on the New Architectural Concept, or Dynamics and Function', Lecture given in Amsterdam, 1923.
11. Tisdall and Bozzolla, 'Futurism and Women', in Futurism, op cit.
12. The tower itself is built of brick covered in stucco due to the shortage of concrete after the First World War.
13. Though confusingly, yet typically, Mendelsohn claimed that the idea of the Einstein Tower came to him while listening to the Christian canticle, the Magnificat. Many of his sketches were inspired by classical composers such as Bach.
14. TS Eliot *Selected Essays*, Faber & Faber (London), 1951.
15. Oskar Beyer, *Letters of an Architect*, Abelard-Schuman (London, New York and Toronto), 1967.

Hermeticism, alchemy and the occult, including witchcraft, rather than Christian morality.[13] We interpret virtue in the sense of power, erotic power and erotic imaginings. Dionysian and tragic indeed. We recall Euripides' play *The Bacchae*, where the arrogant and presumptuous Pentheus is torn limb from limb by the orgiastic and intoxicated forces of Bacchus or Dionysus. In modern literature, Dionysus haunts the ending of F Scott Fitzgerald's *The Great Gatsby* (1925), with its sonorous invocation of an 'orgastic future', of the polymorphous perverse sexuality that provides the erotic underlife to the technological overlife of our century. But in the Einstein Tower, the underlife becomes dominant and subsumes the technology.

Though the shift to eroticism and sensuality took place, architecture has only occasionally responded to Mendelsohn's lead. Frank Lloyd Wright's Johnson Wax factory (1936–9) and the Guggenheim Museum (1942), Le Corbusier's chapel of Ronchamp (1950–54), Jorn Utzon's Sydney Opera House (1956–66) and Frank Gehry's Bilbao Museum (1994–7): a mere handful of virtuous buildings, all of which, including the Einstein Tower, are essentially points of pilgrimage or work. None of them connect with the greatest challenge for architecture, that of housing.

architecture we might say; a cutting edge that saves lives! The whole is full of humour, delight and energy; we feel stimulated and uplifted. As with the Einstein Tower, structure and pleasurable form, Apollo and Dionysus, collaborate in a building that represents the desire for harmony in life, the search for that armistice between the intellect and the senses that lies at the heart of tragedy.

TS Eliot argued in his essay 'The Metaphysical Poets', that it was the dissociation of sensibility associated with the division of the arts and sciences in the 17th century that has led to modern anxieties and feelings of alienation.[14] Prior to that division, as can be seen from the archaic sense of 'virtue', the language of science, alchemy, and poetry were one and the same. Mere poetic metaphors from our erotic vocabulary, for example, 'magnetic attraction', were once thought to signify absolute relations of similitude. Modernism's early project, in poetry, in painting and sculpture was to heal that wound. The Futurists, for example, sensed the energy, the spirit, inherent in all matter or *materia*. They sought a return to the medieval, Thomist world of sacred energy. Mendelsohn – the Nietzschean, German Futurist – wanted to reconnect architecture with the human body in this Dionysian way, recognising that it was the denial of eroticism implied in Apollonian rectilinearity that had led to the orgies of violence and blood lust he had experienced in the First World War and

---

Cascades is a challenging, provocative and ambiguous building. Its pyramidal half-section of Pharaonic burial chambers – machines to speed dead pharaohs on their way to eternity – appears to reincarnate the Thames as a modern Nile.

In recent years, the only example of a virtuous tower dedicated to housing is Rex Wilkinson of CZWG's *Cascades* project (1987–8) in London's Docklands. *Cascades* is a challenging, provocative and ambiguous building. Its pyramidal half-section of Pharaonic burial chambers – machines to speed dead pharaohs on their way to eternity – appears to reincarnate the Thames as a modern Nile. But it is actually a *machine à habiter*. Round porthole windows on the side of the building and ventilation shafts at the front, 'bird's nest' balconies, all indicate naval associations, but dizzyingly, intoxicatingly, the glazed roof of the fire escape reminds one of a guillotine – at the cutting edge of modern

which he wrote about to his wife Louise at the time.[15]

When we experience virtue in architecture, as when we experience it in great literature, painting, music and sculpture, we relax mentally and physically, our arteries and veins expand, our pulse slows and softens, our mind moves freely and imaginatively; we become attuned to the infinite richness of our universe, we become better, energy flows easily through us. *Mens sana in corpore sano*. Great art and architecture, as Aristotle said in the *Poetics*, is cathartic. That restoration of harmony and balance is the purpose of tragedy, but the purpose also of all great art, music and architecture. It incorporates everything, denies nothing. It is virtuous. △

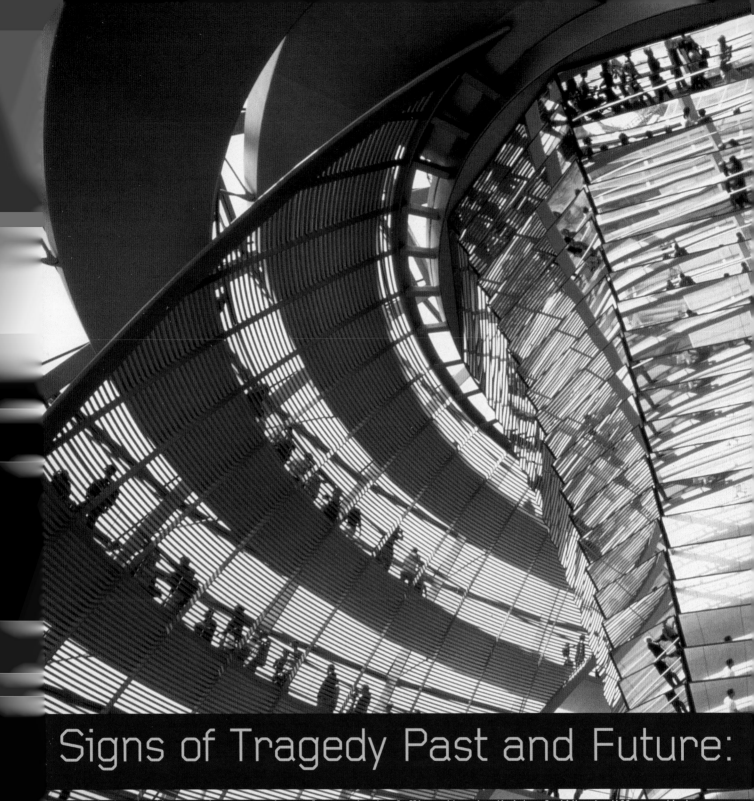

Signs of Tragedy Past and Future:

Tragedy is, in the main, a series of events befalling the individual. What differentiates it from mere disaster is the unknowing collusion of the intentions of the heroic will with sinister fate. It is only in the modern world, with the increase in communication and popular knowledge, that ordinary people have become sufficiently aware of events in the larger context to assume personal responsibility for history. As participants in

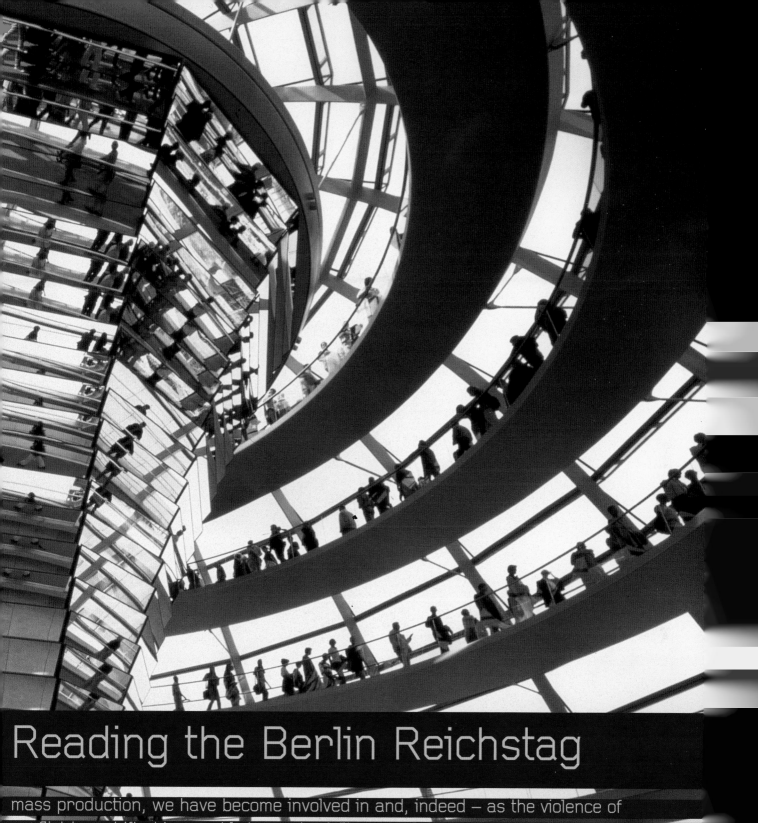

Reading the Berlin Reichstag

mass production, we have become involved in and, indeed – as the violence of conflict has shifted inexorably towards civilian populations – responsible for, actions of state. Tim Martin explores the playing out of the German 'tragedy', illustrating his argument by way of the various phases in the life of the Reichstag in Berlin.

Now that several years have passed since the completion of Norman Foster's work on the Reichstag, there is an opportunity to reflect on the way in which this most allegorical of buildings has settled into Berlin's rapidly growing architectural tapestry. The important question in this case is whether the recent restoration and reconstruction have changed the meaning of the tragic events associated with this building. The Reichstag has provided a stage for so many tragic episodes that it calls out for continued interpretation.

The Reichstag has long been a complex architectural sign in German history. As the first permanent home of a unified national parliament, it was completed in 1882 to a Neo-High Renaissance design at the instigation of Kaiser Wilhelm I. From the day of its opening, it was the home of a weak and fragmented parliament, whose power was resented and distrusted by the militaristic Kaiser Wilhelm II. Though Bismarck preferred a British architect, an all-German competition led to the appointment of Paul Wallot. And though the brief called for a German national style, the classically inspired design was felt to be suitable as an expression of the parliament's position as a powerful component of the German empire. Classical architecture referenced the civic virtues of ancient Rome, and a balance of proportion as a metaphor for a balance of power. The building itself helped structure the political field, assuming power and the existence of other powers.

Almost immediately, a dispute arose over the allegorical meaning of the design. The cupola, meant to symbolise the power of the Kaiser over the legislature was regarded by Wilhelm II as an overbold proclamation of parliamentary power. This power struggle continued over the pediment inscription suggested by the architect: *Dem Deutschen Volke* or 'For the German People'. This was meant to assert the kaiser's gift of the building, and thus his power, but the kaiser chose to exercise his power by forbidding the inscription in order to diminish the parliament's legitimisation. This simultaneously denied imperial and parliamentary power, but seemed wise, nevertheless, since any sign of power relations was bound to be a hostage to future fortunes. Such a sign of imperial power could, after all, be castrated or effaced in favour of the parliament. The blankness of the pediment was thus a sign of uncomfortable power relations until the First World War, when the parliament legitimated itself by ordering the inscription,

which incongruously subordinated it to the emperor. This was feasible because, at this time, the Reichstag had become the place in which Germans gathered to support or protest the war. The kaiser's palace was simply ignored as a site of power.

Power relations worsened under Hitler until the Reichstag was rendered physically dysfunctional by a famously mysterious fire in 1933. While Fascists and Communists blamed each other, Hitler used the fire as a pretext to declare martial law and totalitarian rule. Thus the signs of burning in this building reference a sequence of events in which the loss of an ideal heroic architectural form quickly led to dictatorship. Once the parliament had been stripped of its tectonic cover as symbol of balanced civic responsibility, it was easily rendered politically dysfunctional. Thus the fire proved to be the opening act of the Second World War.

Twelve years later, in the closing act of the war, advancing Soviet troops took Wallot's pediment inscription quite literally, considering the building to be the spatial centre of communal German command, the centre from which National Socialist demands were made and in which satisfaction and pleasure took place. Though empty, it was a prime goal of the assault on Berlin, the many inscriptions on the interior walls left by Soviet troops testifying to its great symbolic importance in the Western world. Despite Hitler's abuse of the building, the gutted and bombed remains became a symbol of the nation to the rest of the world. This much has not changed.

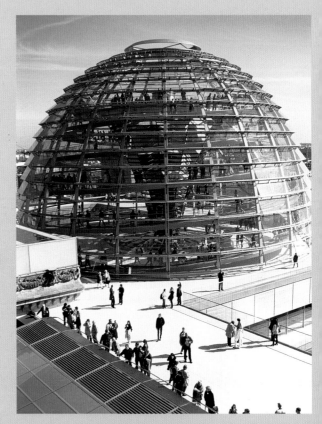

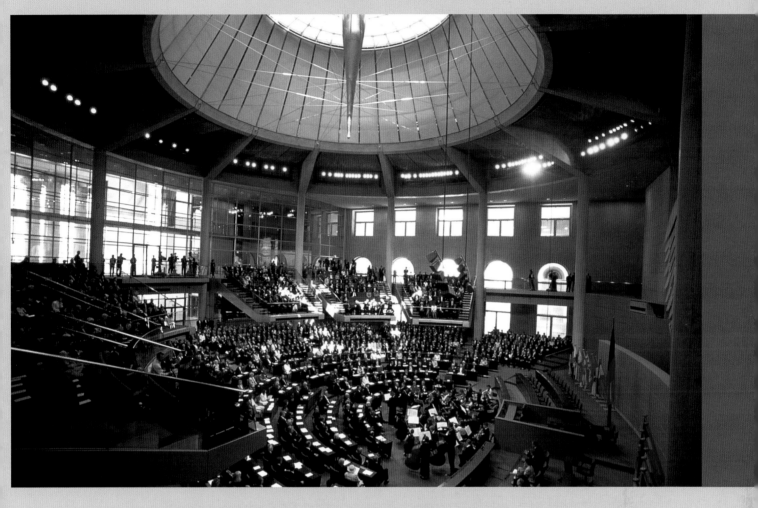

Although it would have been relatively easy, at no point after the Second World War was a decision taken to demolish the outer edifice. Throughout the height of the Cold War, it overlooked the Berlin wall in a state of relative dereliction. Still appropriate in its monumental classical vocabulary, it stood as an empty shell and one of Europe's most haunting of buildings. Its four towers, symbolising the four German kingdoms, acted as a poignantly empty metaphor of national unity and the impossibility of peace in Europe, while a Communist regime ruled East Germany. In this sense, Chancellor Kohl's preference in favour of restoration to original use tends to make the building a symbol of the errors of Fascist and Communist totalitarianism, rather than the failures of communal responsibility.

After reunification, the Reichstag's ghostly presence was emphasised and exorcised in the summer of 1995 when the artists Christo and Jeanne-Claude wrapped the entire, black-streaked pile with white fabric and ropes. This gesture turned the building into a large blank screen, the better to see the powerful symbolic

meanings that were projected on to it by the collective imagination. The terrible memories evoked by the building were for a moment erased, preparing it for a new projection of imagination, and for its once and future role as the locus of communal German power. Had this been a story from an allegorical novel, it might have emerged from its wrapping in its restored and transformed state. As it was, Foster and Partners began work shortly afterwards.

While Foster's restoration was appropriately subtle and minimal in leaving untouched the Cyrillic graffiti and the pediment inscription, other parts of the project entailed wholly new construction and major engineering works. Included in this is a connection to a large water store deep beneath the building, employed to reduce energy consumption. Visually, the most symbolic part of Foster's additions is the new dome, which caps the centre of the building and lies directly over the new debating chamber. While the original cupola was meant to symbolise the kaiser's position at the apex of his empire, as a contemporary political symbol the new dome marks the tenure of Chancellor Kohl. Though now disgraced by scandal, he is the only postwar European leader to realise his major political aspirations, from the unification of Germany under a constitutional

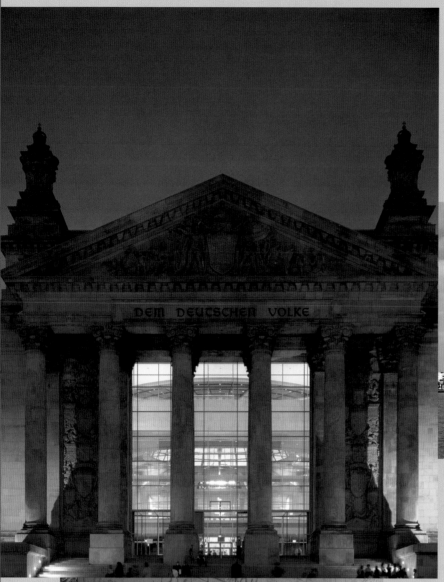

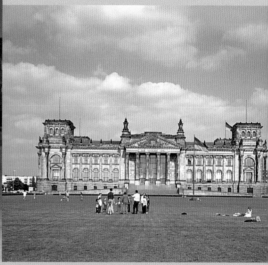

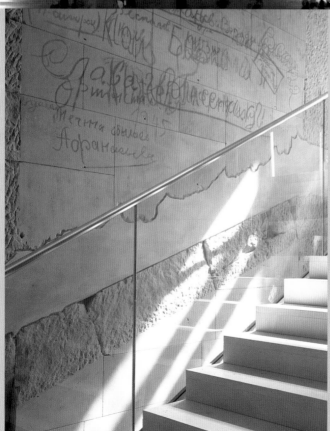

democracy to the institution of a European currency. With Kohl's mark on this building, as with the kaiser's, there is an irony of its 'gift' status, enhanced this time by Christo's giftwrapping. One Foster partner described the dome as 'communicating externally the themes of lightness, transparency, permeability and public access'. That is to say, it reads like a political allegory of Kohl's ideal of government and statesmanship.

The new dome sits higher on the building than the old cupola, and is made from a glazed steel frame to admit light into the building. To enhance the lighting and save energy, a giant conical mirror is suspended in the middle. Its hollow shape also ventilates the chamber. Two helical ramps inside the dome allow large numbers of visitors to observe the parliament below. Interestingly, these ramps are more about satisfying the eye than the ear. They encourage passing observation rather than prolonged listening.

The symbolism of the dome is varied. It has been the subject of many cartoons in the German press, often rendered it as a human part: an eye, a breast, buttocks, etc. In respect of the eye, it recalls the optimised functional visuality of the British panopticon prison: one spectator/warden can keep an eye on all the parliamentarians/prisoners. During the opening ceremony even the leader of the house joked that the visual form of the dome was suited to a paranoiac conception of power. The dome's helical ramps provided Germans with the opportunity to see their government 'from above rather than from below'. In this sense, the dome is an allegory of the eye. From the chamber floor it is the curious conical mirrors that give the slightly paranoid impression of a glinting, watching eye.

In architecture, as elsewhere, there is an attitude toward technology and the machine that calls for its insertion on the site of a trauma. The Reichstag is just such a traumatic site, a tragic backdrop to the parliament; now capped by a symbolic machine. It is an efficient functional device. It is partly a sign of Kohl's political values, partly a reminder of the antitotalitarian structure of democracy in which the government is a servant of the people, and it partly bears a trace of the paranoid eye cast over this building by an authoritarian Kaiser and a Fascist dictator. Metaphorically, the dome invites the world to

also risk becoming a Mannerist device that dissipates the building's tragic form. Equally, the Holocaust Museum now tends to siphon off the Reichstag's tragic associations, leaving behind a structure designed to be appropriate to rational political discourse. The beauty of the Reichstag's functionalist dome is greatest and most stark when experienced in relation to the slashed walls and dissected layout of the Holocaust Museum. Beautifully functional as the dome may be, it is the remaining tragic symbolism in the Reichstag that gives the contemporary German parliament its tectonic structure.

The theatrical grandeur of the dome raises many possibilities. It complements the heroic exuberance of the High Renaissance facade of Wallot, yet it also breaks with its symbolism. The Reichstag is no longer a tragic site for kaiser or dictator to build and destroy. The structure pacifies these battles of political will by placing the German people at its apex. Though this may be read as an allegory of Chancellor Kohl's political values, it also repeats the civic sentiment of Wallot's pediment inscription. With the new dome, the tragic

In architecture, as elsewhere, there is an attitude toward technology and the machine that calls for its insertion on the site of a trauma. The Reichstag is just such a traumatic site.

In architecture, as elsewhere, there is an attitude toward technology and the machine that calls for its insertion on the site of a trauma. The Reichstag is just such a traumatic site.

enter, and now stands in contradistinction to the forbidden central space of Libeskind's Holocaust Museum.

After the fall of the wall, but before the completion of this museum, the Reichstag was alone in Berlin in being an architecture of tragic form and proportion. The devastation of the building, and its traumatic symbolism required resolution within the building rather than within the city. Perhaps for this reason, Foster sought to include powerful lamps that would illuminate the inside of the dome and radiate outward. Working with a New York stage-lighting designer, Foster experimented with the number and aim of the beams. At night, the dome can now be turned into a twelve-bulbed 'lighthouse' that emits a constant horizontal array of light, which seeks to be a positive metaphor of the civic duties and rights of parliamentary democracy. It would be the closing act of the tragedy, the point at which interpretation and meaning is invited. Whether a piece of uncritical triumphalism to make Albert Speer envious, or a somewhat theatrical party trick on the theme of Fritz Lang's *Metropolis*, the illuminations can

is formed in a different way from in the past. While, in the day, the dome pacifies the tragedy wrought by 20th-century ideological excess, on some nights the lighthouse effect takes over. With this shift, the dome conspicuously consumes the electrical power that it meticulously saves in the day. It acts as a metaphoric guide, a beacon of rational political measure and limit. In effect, it acts like the final scene of a tragedy in which resolution is reached. As it streaks through the city, though, its light can turn slightly more sinister, seeming like an inescapable and unrestrained eye. It exceeds urban limits, aspires to expand indefinitely, to see and illuminate beyond its scope. In short, it has a paranoiac structure for some, as evidenced in the jokes that have appeared in the press.

These are relative readings, when in fact the lighthouse may be too contradictory and theatrical to be part of a clear symbolic moral. The dome's lighthouse effect is a question of decorum, of getting the right balance between modesty and grandeur. Yet it inevitably suggests future tragedy, without pointing in any one direction. If it hints at anything in the night, it is of a communal dream of environmental tragedy, and of the return of crimes committed, oddly enough, in the name of functionalism and efficiency. Δ

Opposite top left
The west entry at dusk, showing the pediment inscription, which was retained in Foster's subtle treatment of the parliament building.

Opposite top right
The Reichstag in Berlin, in 1992, before renovation.

Opposite bottom
Interior detail of Foster & Partners' new restoration of the Bundestag. Above the stairs, the Cyrillic graffiti are left bare.

The Metamorphosis

The term 'tragedy' has transmuted from its precise classical sense to become a general handbag containing any meanings concerned with personal frustration and loss. Richard Patterson traces its vicissitudes from the Greek literary genre into the modern. He argues that the basic framework it established was essential to the Western visual tradition and that its legacy remains a determining factor in the structure of Western cultural production.

# of Tragedy

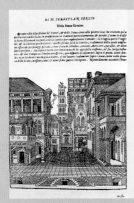
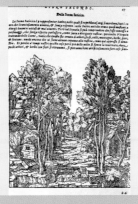
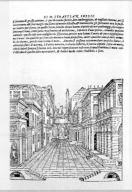

Tragedy and Symbolic Representation

In his taxonomic scenes of tragedy, comedy and the satyric, Sebastiano Serlio provides us with the clearest representation of these genres in Renaissance architecture. This taxonomy is derived from Vitruvius 5.6.9:

> the tragic is represented by columns and pediments and figures and other regal things ... the Comic by private and meandering buildings ... the Satyric will be equipped with trees, caves, mountains and other rustic things represented in the shapes of garden topiary.

These lines were to have a profound effect on propriety in Renaissance architecture and garden design. But the genres were derived from the literary, dramatic and narrative tradition as delineated by Aristotle, for example in the opening lines of the *Poetics:*

> Epic poetry and Tragedy, Comedy also, Dithyrambic poetry, and the music of the flute and of the lyre in most of their forms, are all in their general conception modes of imitation. They differ, however, from one another in three respects, the medium, the objects, the manner or mode of imitation, being in each case distinct.

With Serlio, we need only invoke Horace's dictum *ut pictura poesis* in order to discern the medium, the objects, and the manner and mode of imitation of the architectural genres. The comic scene is unremarkable, disorderly and domestic – these are buildings, but there is no consistency in style or application. The satyric is little more than trees, raw, natural and unbounded. But the tragic was to be made of Architecture: proper, civic, urban Architecture. At the centre of the scene, for example, there is a church facade that reminds us of a tradition of Renaissance design that began with Alberti's facade to Santa Maria Novella, Florence. There are correctly disposed buildings, set in a regular

formal composition, ready to accommodate all the functions of state. The designation of this scene as 'tragic' is premised on the criteria of that genre as described by Aristotle.

To begin with, Aristotle's discussion of the genres reflects certain primary classical models. The principle of tradition and the act of emulation as the fundamental resources from which the poet derives his work are universal. The nature of the poet's work is to be found in the twin acts of selection and combination. Working in a known framework, propriety or judgement was a fundamental responsibility for the poet. Each genre demanded the selection of a correct level of language; it required the judicious selection of incidents – terms and so on – and a certain propriety in their combination into the structure of the text. Each genre that one might wish to emulate had its distinct objective, and its specific form.

Even amongst this seemingly neutral set of types, tragedy had a special place. It was the most highly developed; it had a historical origin; it was the most recent; it was engaged in theoretical questions of historical significance. It has been said of Sophocles that historically and conceptually he occupies a median position between 'rootedness in archaic ideals ... and that move towards bathos, sentimentality, criticism and sophistry' that we associate with narcissistic individualism and self-consciousness.[1] Tragedy appeared at a crucial period of transformation in Greek history. We know from Aristotle that it had been developed from epic and the dithyramb, just as comedy had originated in lampooning and phallic songs.[2] It had to work within an explicit framework and, unlike epic, was only allowed a single plot, which had to be completed within a limited period: the circuit of a single sun, or one day. Most importantly, it had to be 'an imitation of an action complete and whole ... by language that (had) been artificially enhanced by rhythm and song'.[3] This idea of the whole, moreover, was not merely a stylistic, expressive unity. It was in fact the 'plot' bounded by critical breaks in the chain of causality.

Left
Sebastiano Serlio, 'comic scene', *Tutte l'Opere D'Architettura, et Prospetiva* Venice (G de'Franceschi 1619, p 45v).

Middle
Sebastiano Serlio, 'satyric scene', *Tutte l'Opere D'Architettura, et Prospetiva* Venice (G de'Franceschi 1619, p 47r).

Right
Sebastiano Serlio, 'tragic scene', *Tutte l'Opere D'Architettura, et Prospetiva* Venice (G de'Franceschi 1619, p 46v).

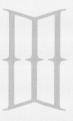

Tragedy is the primordial form of poetry in which there is a measurable limit. It introduces the concept of limit for a text, a means, thereby, for turning actions into texts, and making them things.

Aristotle said:

'A whole is that which has a beginning, a middle, and an end. A beginning is that which does not itself follow anything by causal necessity, but after which something naturally is or comes to be. An end, on the contrary, is that which itself naturally follows some other thing, either by necessity, or as a rule, but has nothing following it. A middle is that which follows something as some other thing follows it.'[4]

Tragedy is the primordial form of poetry in which there is a measurable limit. It introduces the concept of limit for a text, a means, thereby, for turning actions into texts, and making them things. Time can be our first marker of the tragic. The principle of a temporal unity underwrites the concept of tragedy. An action bounded by time is thereby a whole action; it has a certain 'objectness' about it. Time and action, time and motion; the first strategic trope of the tragic is reification.

The reference to Alberti as the originator of one of the forms in Serlio's engraving is not fortuitous, for it would barely be an exaggeration to claim that the history of the visual arts in the West is but a series of footnotes to Alberti. The *De re aedificatoria* (1452), his treatise on architecture, set our theoretical basis for reflective practice in building. In the *De pictura* (1436), he set out the theoretical principle of *compositio*, by which he meant a four-level hierarchy of forms running from planes (of colour), to members, to bodies, to the *historia*, from form to action.[5] Michael Baxandall has written of Alberti's use of medieval rhetorical treatises in the formulation of this principle, in the use of an arborescent order, as the invocation of an essentially literary authority for the linking of textual unity with action.[6] Alberti's criterion for wholeness was ultimately Aristotelian; its standard was Ciceronian:

'that no part might be added or taken away but to the detriment of the whole.'[7]

It set a new standard of specificity for visual composition – that of the plot, so to speak, the *historia* as a causal necessity, a temporal specificity, and an 'organic' unity, which effectively established the tragic as the grounding of proper visual composition up to the 19th century.[8]

There was no equivalent for the other genres, for comedy or for the *satyric* for the simple reason that these parts of the *Poetics* had been lost. The form of the tragic became the basis of æsthetic theory, in part at least, because it was available. Which is not to say that discursive, irregular, iconographic programmes were entirely superseded by the advent of Renaissance classicism, but rather that they were beyond the purview of theory or criticism.[9] Narrative, as a form of recording or ritual, no longer held sway over the totalising imperatives of form. Conceptualising this transformation can be achieved by returning to the Aristotelian framework.

Tragedy, according to Aristotle, differs from history, in the sense that whereas history deals with something that has happened (and may be episodic), tragedy deals with interpretation, the perception and consciousness of actions that might happen or might have happened. It concerns intention, perception, error and psychic reconciliation. Tragedy structures a threshold between three things: what is really going on, but is unnoticed; the imaginary world of the subject's narcissistic identity; and symbolic representation. Aristotle makes this threshold event clear in the requirement he placed on the structure of the plot: the reversal of the situation, the recognition (that is to say, that moment of the awakening of perception into consciousness, that moment at which material signs become symbols, enter discourse and acquire significance) and the scene of suffering. The price of catharsis is destructive or painful acts, bodily agony and 'wounds' – in the Greek, *trauma*.[10]

So, 'Tragedy is an imitation not only of a complete action, but of events inspiring fear or pity.' The inspiration of fear and pity in the observer, that is, who

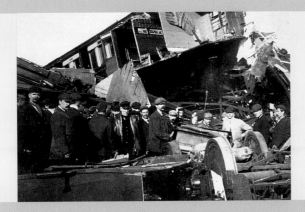

by way of a judgement that 'what has happened is manifestly possible', may be ensnared through projective identification into the plot and its consequences.[11] But the aim of tragedy, according to Aristotle, is actually the reverse: that is, a movement beyond the traumatic event to the purgation of 'fear and pity'. It is in this principle that Lacan finds 'the true significance of tragedy ... with the excitement involved, in connection with the emotions ... with the singular emotions of fear and pity', the dissipation of the order of the imaginary, the purgation of the imaginary by fear and pity. 'It has to do', he claims, 'with the intervention of beauty ... and with the place (that beauty) occupies between two fields that are symbolically differentiated.'[12] This moment of transfer between symbolic regimes (if we allow Lacan's terminology), between the narcissistic regime of the imaginary and the desire for the symbolic other, is, observed Aristotle, to be 'best produced when the events come on us by surprise; and the effect is heightened when, at the same time, they follow as cause and effect', that is, when the observer is captured within the chain of causation.

Trauma and Mechanisation

The significance of tragedy, as we have noted, lies in the dissipation of the imaginary and the reassertion of the symbolic. But what happens if the action is not whole, if the imaginary is confounded, say; if, using another set of terms, when the imaginary unity of narcissistic identification is disturbed there is no moment of identification with the beautiful; no consciousness, that is, of the grounds of our most profound anxiety? We know, of course, the name of the discourse that has historically addressed this condition, this deferred resolution, this foreclosure. Since the 18th century, it has been called *the sublime*. For Kant, the sublime articulated a 'lack of fit' between the subject and nature, a lack of fit that he saw as the basis of personal freedom. For Burke, the sublime simply signified a failure of the subject, a failure to render sensation as cognition. Sublime themes concern the infinite and the violent, anything that the mind cannot symbolise, anything that is radically resistant to consciousness and to language; anything that 'exceeds cognition'.

Throughout the 19th century, there is a persistent development of themes of the sublime, either natural, as we are familiar with in the violence of Landseer 'nature red in tooth and claw', in the anomalies of classification and identity in freak shows, or man made, in the form of a growing morbid interest in mechanised or industrial catastrophe. This is the moment when the principle of the tragic ceased to sustain discourse, when the possibility of symbolic representation was foreclosed, when tragedy became the question that 'cannot be answered.'

Until the 19th century, 'trauma' was used to refer simply to 'wounds' or the 'cure of wounds'. By mid-century, however, it had come to be used by way of reference to a mental wound. Originally thought to have been caused by 'powerful blows or shocks ... or concussions of the spinal cord' that had not left visible evidence, mental trauma could be blamed on almost anything, including surgical operations or injuries in general. But the paradigm case of all such speculation was railway accidents. John Erichsen wrote in 1866:

'In no ordinary accident, can the shock be so great as those that occur on Railways. The rapidity of the movement, the momentum of the person injured, the suddenness of arrest, the helplessness of the sufferers, and that natural perturbation of mind that must disturb the bravest, are all circumstances that of necessity increase the severity of the resulting injury to the nervous system.'[13]

Following this medical topos, Freud using another set of terms later raised issues of warfare and mechanisation in what would be his first analysis of a form of trauma that was neither explicitly sexual nor, for that matter, even personal. In *Beyond the Pleasure*

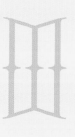
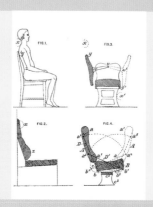
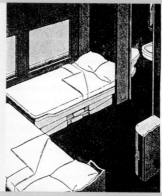
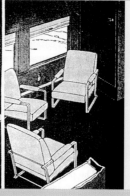
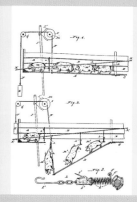

Principle (1920), he wrote:

> A condition has been known and described
> which occurs after several mechanical
> concussions, railway disasters and other
> accidents involving a risk to life; it has been
> given the name of 'traumatic neurosis'. The
> terrible war which has just ended gave rise
> to a great number of illnesses of this kind,
> but it at least put an end to the temptation to
> attribute the cause of the disorder to organic
> lesions of the nervous system brought about
> by mechanical force.[14]

The disallowance of physical contact from the
necessary aetiology of this traumatic malady
underlines Freud's interpretation of the
condition's purely psychic character. Further on
in the same piece he even noted 'that a wound
or injury inflicted simultaneously works as a rule
against the development of (such) a neurosis'.[15]
For Freud then, as for Aristotle, the physical
trauma was but a visual metaphor, a tropic
fulcrum, if you will, of psychic impact and
transformation. And for Freud, the traumatic
neurosis was more likely to be visited upon the
observer than the victim. In this context, Freud
was explicit about the role of symbolic discourse
in achieving psychic closure:

> Artistic play and artistic imitation carried out
> by adults unlike children's (play), are aimed at
> an audience, and do not spare the spectators
> (for instance, in tragedy) the most painful
> experiences and can yet be felt by them as
> highly enjoyable.[16]

If, however, action exceeds or evades symbolic
representation, the possibility of closure is,
as it were, foreclosed, and the subject is
overwhelmed, 'traumatised' and forced into a
neurotic structure. The ego may be restructured
around a question and the incident rendered
inaccessible to symbolic representation.

Siegfried Giedion, long established as one of
the major apologists for modernism, mounted an
unintentional exploration of the twin themes of
modernity and trauma in *Mechanization Takes
Command* (1948).[17] I say 'unintentional' because his
argument, while intuitively strong, is by our standards
inadequately theorised. For one thing, he never
mentioned trauma, but he did state his intention as
follows:

> In *Space, Time and Architecture* (1941), I attempted
> to show the split that exists in our period between
> thought and feeling. I am trying now to go a step
> further: to show how this break came about, by
> investigation of one important aspect of our life –
> mechanization.[18]

Whilst his definition of 'mechanization' is often
reasonable enough ('the end product of a rationalistic
view of the world', the dissection of 'work into its
component operations' and, after Adam Smith, the
'division of labour'), and he notes that 'all aspects
of life have been inextricably interwoven with it', he is
nonetheless only able to offer an undefined 'organic
unity' to oppose it.[19]

His themes are moreover curious and fetishistic –
he seems to avoid the obvious. There is, curiously, no
section specifically on transportation, the section on
'Railroads and Patent Furniture' being concerned with
cataloguing modes of interface between human bodies
and mechanical systems. There is similarly no section
on architecture: that on the 'household' is limited to
electrical and mechanical appliances. But there is a
section where he actually approaches the question of
feeling (and where he writes the most poetic material
in the whole of his *oeuvre*) entitled 'Mechanization and
Organic Substance', and most direct in this regard is
the chapter 'Mechanization and Death: Meat'.

This is the section in which he famously researched
the historical origin of assembly-line production in the
slaughterhouses of the Chicago stockyards. He wrote:

> It was through the whole method behind (the)
> process (of mechanized meat production) that the
> assembly line came about. In the packing industry ...
> decades of assembly-line experience were gained.
> The automobile industry was able to work out its own

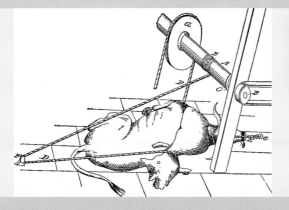

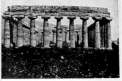

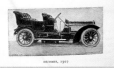

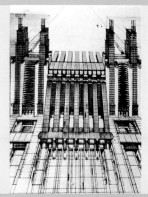

assembly line with such astonishing speed because of the extensive practice gained here in working on the moving object.[20]

But, far from a paean to modernism, what follows is an extraordinary description of the paradigmatic deadness of mechanised production, of the mechanical violence of its endless repetition, of action, that is, committed outside the framework of symbolic discourse:

> In one of the great packing plants, an average of two animals are killed every second … The death cries of the animals whose jugular veins have been opened are confused with the rumbling of the great drum, the whirring of gears, and the shrilling sound of steam. Death cries and mechanical noises are almost impossible to disentangle. Neither can the eye quite take in what it sees. On one side of the sticker are the living; on the other side, the slaughtered. Each animal hangs head downwards at the same regular interval, except that, from the creatures to his right, blood is spurting out of the neck-wound in the tempo of the heart beat. In twenty seconds, on the average, a hog is supposed to have bled to death. It happens so quickly, and is so smooth a part of the production process, that emotion is barely stirred.

And in the following there is one of the most poignant descriptions of post traumatic stress disorder that I have ever read:

> …what is truly startling in this mass transition from life to death is the complete neutrality of the act. One does not experience, one does not feel; one merely observes. It may be that nerves that we do not control rebel somewhere in the subconscious. Days later, the inhaled odour of blood suddenly rises from the walls of one's stomach, although no trace of it can have clung to the person.[21]

But curiously, despite this rhetoric, there is no mention in Giedion of warfare despite, one

suspects, the fact that warfare was the origin of these literary conceits. Perhaps this is the point. Perhaps this is the very point of the aesthetics of modernity: that by maintaining a certain segregation of topics according to various discourses (either of trauma or of beauty), we are able to figure a defensive repression of some of the more potent anxieties of our time.

The Machine Aesthetic

'The machine aesthetic' is a modernist term variously used to refer to the forms, mode of production and psychically dislocating abstractions of mechanisation. It has been a significant rallying cry for art and architecture throughout the modernist epoch. Repeatedly, this aesthetic has proposed a new form of optical vision arising from the objective mentality of the engineer. That is, an aesthetic mentality that might actually calculate its compositions 'machine-like' such, 'that no part might be added or taken away but to the detriment of the whole'. But in this new 20th-century invocation of Cicero, it is not the elegance of the syllogism that is taken to mean beauty, but a mechanistic determinism.

Historically, the machine aesthetic began with Marinetti's prologue to his 'foundation manifesto', which was published in *Le Figaro* on 20 February 1909. It is a model of the catechretic application of a mode of discourse, a genre, to inappropriate objects and actions. It exemplifies the expropriation of the discourse of beauty as a eulogy to the sublime. Rayner Banham has said of the prologue that it 'mimic(s) a baptism in Jordan … into the experiences and mental categories of mechanical sensibility'.[22]

> I swung the car round in its own length, like a mad dog trying to bite its own tail … I pulled up so short that the car … looped into the ditch and came to rest with its wheels in the air.
> O maternal ditch, brimming with muddy water –
> O factory drain! I gulped down your nourishing mud and … yet, when I emerged … I felt the hot iron of a delicious joy in my heart.[23]

And the juxtaposition of classical references with

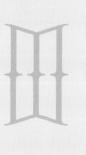

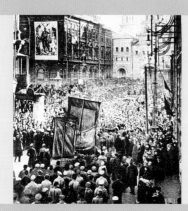

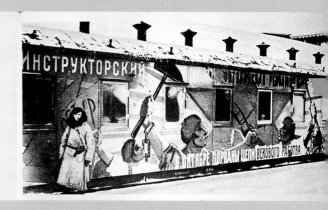

Notes
1. Jacques Lacan, *The Ethics of Psychoanalysis*, Tavistock/ Routledge (London), 1992, p 273.
2. Aristotle, *Poetics*, Bk IV.
3. Ibid, Bk VI, 4–12.
4. Ibid, Bk VII.
5. Leon Battista Alberti, *On Painting and On Sculpture: the Latin texts of De picture and De statua*, ed and trans Cecil Grayson, Phaidon Press (London), 1972, p 21.
6. Michael Baxandall *Giotto and the Orators*, Clarendon Press (Oxford), 1971, pp 130–31; for a discussion of the Vitruvian basis, via Barbaro, of a 'linguistic' basis for the visual tradition see Oskar Batschmann, 'Diskurs der Architektur im Bild' in Carlpeter Braegger (ed), *Architektur und Sprache* Prestel-Verlag, (Munich), 1982: See Caroline van Eck 'Enduring Principles of Architecture in Alberti's On the Art of Building: how did Alberti set out to formulate them?', *The Journal of Architecture*, vol 4/2 (1999), pp 119–29.
7. The principle is a traditional one and occurs in Cicero's *De oratore*, Bk III.viii.29 in a speech referring to Catullus: 'What greater treat have our ears had than the eloquence of our friend Catullus? Its style is so pure that he seems almost the only person that speaks sound Latin ... when listening to him my regular verdict is that any addition or alteration or subtraction you might make would be inferior – an alteration for the worse'.
8. See Svetlana Alpers, *The Art of Describing: Dutch Art in the Seventeenth Century*,

machine technology is even more overt in the main body of the text:

> We declare that the splendour of the world has been enriched by a new beauty – the beauty of speed. A racing car with its bonnet draped with exhaust pipes like fire-breathing serpents – a roaring racing car, rattling along like a machine gun, is more beautiful than the winged victory of Samothrace.[24]

Marinetti never makes a claim for an intrinsic criteria of beauty in the machine. The catechretic use of beauty in metaphors like 'pipes like fire-breathing serpents', or quantitative phrases ('more beautiful'), and in the parasitic, even kitsch, use of tradition ('the winged victory of Samothrace'), all point to a different agenda, more along the lines, it is my argument, of a defensive repression. Within the community of its production, modernism was indeed subject to the repression of its sublime, traumatic impact under the rubric of the beautiful. Outside the discourse of modernity, outside the community of its production, where modernism's mode of reception was not subject to this discursive repression, the experience of modernity has most frequently been characterised as the 'shock of the new', that is, simply as trauma. [25]

Trauma as Cultural Currency

For the Cubists, the discourse of modernity was focused primarily on the impact of mechanisation on the work of art. For the Futurists it was more ideological, engaging the everyday, extending even to eulogies to war and machine sports. It was only with the Russian Revolution that the power of trauma was recognised and promulgated as a positive vehicle of social transformation. The most extreme versions of this programme can be found in the writings of the Constructivists, in which are outlined the concrete programmatic implications of a Soviet, Marxist revolutionary speculation. In general, Marx had identified the justness of revolution in a structural elimination of the alienation arising from 'exchange value' and its concomitant social forms. He had argued that it would develop into an epitome in consequence of the complete separation of ownership from labour under the capitalist 'mode of production'. According to his model, a continuing condensation of capital would occur until such time as the whole of the working population had become dispossessed, alienated, and no longer in control of their lives or bodies. But far from seeing this as an embodiment of evil Marx held, in an overtly Hegelian sense, that this was a historical, structural necessity for the creation of a revolutionary class, to be called the proletariat. Hypothetically, the proletariat would develop a concept of human universality by virtue of its definitive dispossession of private property and the location of the criteria of its social identity in production alone. To reiterate, from a state of having no control of their lives or bodies, the proletariat would accede to a state of universality and banish alienation definitively.

But the means of production to which Marx referred was mechanised and by the time of the revolution in 1918 it was not sufficiently developed in Russia, which certainly had nothing resembling a significant proletariat. This was, perhaps, the major theoretical problem faced by Lenin, for which he developed the concept of the 'dictatorship of the proletariat' as a mandate for the Communist Party. In the absence of a historically created proletariat it would, accordingly, be the responsibility of the Communist Party to be its agent, and the model Lenin developed for this principle was not that of a representative parliamentary body of government, containing opposition parties and subject to open debate. Rather it was that of the Western bourgeois professional institution with its emphasis on technical standards and ethical behaviour, subject only to independent, internal peer review, interpretation of competence, professional judgement and discipline.

We must now read the theoretical and ideological documents of Russian artists and architects of the revolutionary period in a new light. They were explicitly professional, technical documents, with an explicitly

All images from left to right

1. May Day, 1919
2. Pashkov and Gerasimov: Propaganda Train, 1919–20.
3. Malevitch & Unovis, conference of teachers and students.
4. Rodchenko, Paris Pavilion Workers' Club.
5.1. (below) 'The pleasures of the individual household'.
5.2. (below)'The rationalised laundry in collectivised housing'.

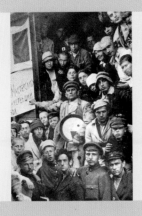

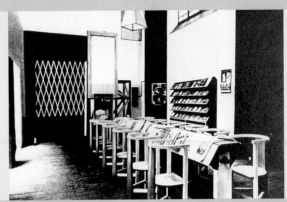

University of Chicago Press (Chicago), 1983; Alpers' distinction between 'Northern' and 'Southern' modes can, I believe, be more critically made by way of a distinction between epic and tragic.
9. Richard Patterson, 'The Hortus Palatinus and the Reformation of the World', *Journal of Garden History*, i, 1 & 2, pp 67–104, 179–202.
10. Aristotle, *Poetics* , Bk XI.
11. Ibid, Bk IX.
12. Lacan, op cit, pp 247–48.
13. John Erichsen, *On Railway and Other Injuries of the Nervous System*, Walton and Maberley (London), 1866, p 9.
14. Sigmund Freud, *Beyond the Pleasure Principle*, reprinted in Peter Gay, *The Freud Reader*, Vintage (London), 1995, vol 3, pp 31–38.
15. Ibid, p 598.
16. Ibid, p 601.
17. Siegfried Giedion, *Mechanization Takes Command*, Oxford University Press (Oxford), 1948.
18. Ibid, pv.
19. There are many examples of naiveté in Giedion's remarks, of which this is perhaps one of the more humorous: 'It need only be added that in manufacturing complex products such as the automobile, this division (of labour) goes together with a reassembly', ibid p 32.
20. Ibid, p 229.
21. Ibid, p 246.
22. Reyner Banham *Theory and Design in the First Machine Age*, Butterworth-Heinemann (Oxford), 1994, p 103.
23. Quoted in ibid, p 102.
24. Ibid, p 103.
25. See my 'Trauma, Modernity and the Sublime', *Journal of Architecture*, Spring 1999.
26. Quoted in Catherine Cooke 'The Development of the Constructivist Architects' Design Method' in A Papadakis, C Cooke and A Benjamin, *Deconstruction Omnibus Volume*, Academy Editions (London), 1989, p 38.

professional mandate: to 'transform a way of life', to create the concrete basis for the realisation of an artificially dispossessed proletariat. In the absence of a proletariat historically realised by the capitalist mode of production, an artificial proletariat might be created by the imposition of the purest, most abstract, de-personalising elements of mechanisation as such. From a poster from the Soviet Institute for Scientific Organisation of Work Processes, which was conducting an overtly Taylorist campaign, this seminal proletariat was exhorted with the words, 'Let us take the storm of the Revolution in Russia and unite it to the pulse of life in America and do our work like a chronometer'.[26] Here, we see fairly clearly how the old bourgeois systems of symbolic domination were to be replaced by the traumatised psyches of the proletariat, under a code of objective, scientific social discourse, as protocyborg extensions of the machine.

The Soviet housing programme is well documented as intending to collectivise dwelling and eliminate the family as the primary living unit. What distinguished this programme from more traditional student, collegiate or monastic forms of collective living, however, was the determination to regulate domestic relations by a formally mechanical 'mode of production'. In a poster advocating collective laundry facilities, there is a clear indication that playing with children during productive domestic work is not correct proletarian behaviour, nor indeed is conversation as we infer from the stance of the women in the mechanised facility. In other words, the Soviet programme took the oxymoron of the 'machine aesthetic' literally, as the formal basis of an Enlightenment project of emancipation.

The historic function of the tragic lay in the quite exquisite structure with which it provided symbolic discourse in the event of individual folly and blind fate. But the tragic is about a closure that has little place in a world of continuous, mechanical production. What is foreclosed in the traumatised observer of that world is what we might refer to as the spiritual, or, to use Aristotle's terminology, the 'recognition', or Lacan's, the 'dissipation' of the imaginary, so that what we are left with is an eternally traumatised, nondiscursive experience of the world. △

This article is based on a paper delivered at the Royal Academy Forum, 'The Tragic in Art and Architecture', in London on 16 March 1999.

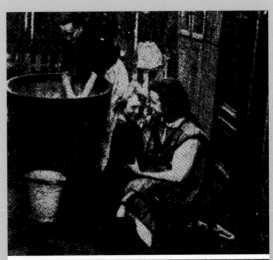

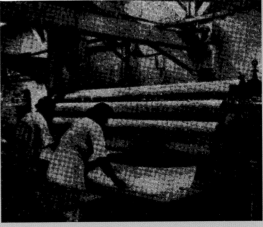

Death in

The Spectre of the Tragic
New Extension to San Mi

The most significant architectural intervention to take place in Venice over the last hu
by approximately 64,500 square metres to receive new structures and freshly laid ou
David Chipperfield Architects, is due on site in the summer of 2001 with the completio
such a spiritually charged and historically poised project might evoke closure in a ma

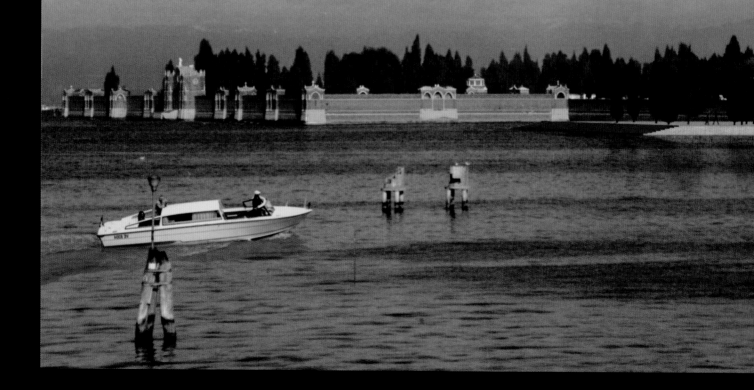

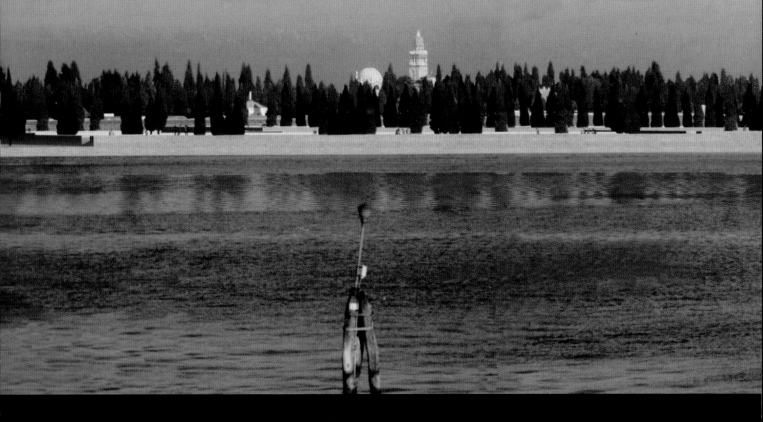

Venice

David Chipperfield's
...ele Cemetery

...ears is currently under way. The cemetery island of San Michele is being extended
...grounds on two lots of reclaimed land. The scheme, which is being developed by
...irst few structures planned for the end of 2001. Here, Helen Castle discusses how
...is in keeping with some of the conventions of classical tragedy.

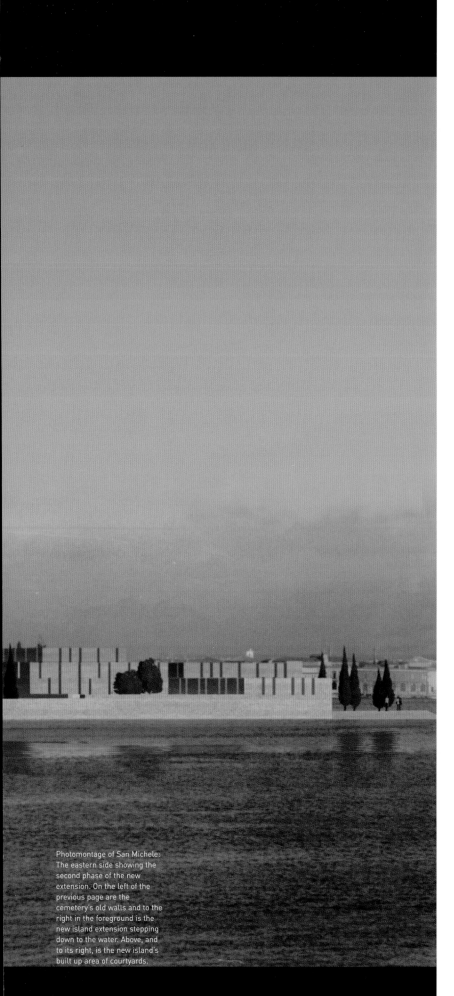

Cemeteries perhaps offer the greatest potential
for the tragic genre. This is not as the
architecture of death per se, but as places of
reconciliation where, often in grief, the living
are forced to confront the mortality of others
and ultimately themselves. As Richard Patterson
points out in his essay in this publication, the
aim of tragedy as outlined by Aristotle is
restorative: 'a movement beyond the traumatic
event to the purgation of "fear and pity".'[1]
In dramatic tragedy this culminates in the final
scene of a play, where resolution generally
follows close on the heels of death.

San Michele Cemetery's unique location
marks it out as a place of quiet and spiritual
restoration. On a small island, no more than
several hundred metres from Venice's northern
shore, it is easily identifiable from land and
sea by its dark cypresses, high 19th-century
brick walls and the gleaming white facade of
its Mauro Coducci church. Lorenzetti describes
the view of the cemetery island from the
Fondamenta Nuove as one of,

> '...tender melancholy. The silence, the
> limitless stretch of water, the view of San
> Michele, the isle of the dead, surrounded by
> the dark mass of cypress trees, all suggest
> to the mind sad thoughts; it is a new
> fascination, different from the usual which
> affects the visitor.'[2]

This 'melancholy fascination' transcends
the humdrum routine of tourist Venice, with its
gondoliers, cheap pizzas and speedy tours of
the Piazza San Marco. It expresses something
about the life and death of native Venetians
– in the present as much as in the past. And
their mindfulness of the departed. The cemetery
is serviced by shops in Venice itself, on the
Fondamenta Nuove the embankment opposite
the island. Stonemasons, flower stalls and shops
selling fabric flowers are clustered around the
Calle de Croci, a signed route leading from the
Rialto to the vaporetto stop for San Michele. With
vaporetti stopping off at the island at 10-minute
intervals, it is an easily reachable haven rather
than an outpost. On a Saturday morning in June,
for instance, you find yourself jostling among
several dozen widows, bearing bouquets, for a
place on board the ferry. Once on the island, the
cemetery is filled with the gentle buzz of people
lovingly tending graves – replacing fresh and
artificial flowers and murmuring prayers.

Ever since 1804, when the first general
cemetery of Venice was established on the island
of San Cristoforo – now adjoined to San Michele
– the cemetery has been the focus of Venetian

civitas or civic pride. (Previous to Napoleon's Edict of St Cloud, which declared all cemeteries should be removed for public health reasons from the centres of towns across Europe, graveyards were attached to local parish churches within the city.) Native Venetians have unceasingly desired to be buried in the city cemetery within Venice's lagoon. From the start, the cemetery has had to be continually enlarged in the effort to keep up with demand. Only three years after the original cemetery on San Cristoforo was completed in 1813 by Giannantonio Selva, plans were being made to extend the burial ground to include the island of San Michele – until then, primarily a Camaldolese monastery. Between 1835 and 1839, the 85 metres of land dividing San Cristoforo from San Michele were reclaimed from the lagoon under the direction of Giuseppe Salvadori. The island was further expanded to the east in the 1840s and the 1860s, when Annibale Forcellini added the distinctive red-brick enclosing wall topped with a *pietra d'Istria* frame. The extension of the burial ground continued into the 20th century with the realisation of a *sacca* along the eastern wall in the first few decades; in 1975, a further *sacca* was established on the northeastern edge to collect mud accumulated from the excavation of canals. Though Venice's permanent population was by this time decreasing, pressure on the cemetery's land never ceased. Even when, after 10 or 12 years, corpses began to be interred in ossuaries, there were still not enough places in the cemetery. In recent years, this situation has been compounded by soil erosion, which has meant corpses have taken longer to decompose in the ground. Increasing numbers have had to be buried at Mestre and in other towns. Throughout, however, Venetians have remained adamant that it is their civic right to be buried at San Michele.

By the late 1990s, the Comunità di Venezia already had plans under way to extend the cemetery. Handled as a municipal works project without any real architectural aspirations, it was to be conducted in a routine manner. The mayor, however, who was unhappy about this process, applied the brakes and invoked the idea of an international architectural competition. Some 150 offices submitted cvs, out of which eight were shortlisted and invited to develop proposals. Half of the final submissions were Italian, and the remaining half from other European countries. The winning entry came from the London-based practice David

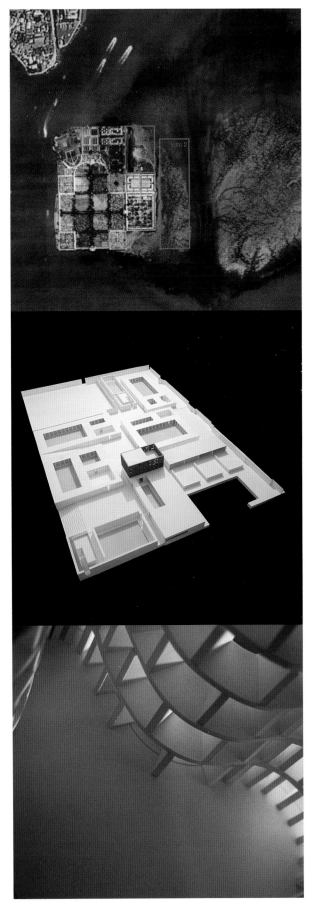

Top
Photomontage of San Michele looking to the south towards Venice, with David Chipperfield Architects' design for the new extension superimposed.

Middle
Model of the first phase of the extension of San Michele, looking south. In the bottom right is a harbour and the cemetery's service areas. In the centre is the building that will take the form of the as yet unfinalised chapel, with the remaining area being given over to courtyards.

Bottom
Model of a proposed design for the chapel on the first phase of the extension. Though unfinalised, Chipperfield Architects are working on the design concept for a chapel that is organic in form and transparent, contrasting with the solidity of the courtyard blocks.

Chipperfield Architects. Without a doubt, Chipperfield's simple, rational and craft-based approach has struck an aesthetic chord with the Italians: in little more than a couple of years, the office has won three out of the five major competitions that it has entered in Italy. These include the Ansaldo 'City of Cultures' museum complex in Milan and the Salerno Palace of Justice. The practice is also architect to the Italian fashion house Dolce & Gabbana, and is presently designing them a whole string of shops worldwide.[3] In Venice, Chipperfield's work has a particular resonance. He works in a similar métier to that of Carlo Scarpa, the only modern architect to make any significant impact on Venice and the Veneto in the 20th century. Chipperfield shares with Scarpa not only a regard for materials, but also a common treatment of space and volume.

It was, nonetheless, the simplicity and clarity of Chipperfield's proposal rather than its detailing or style that recommended it to the jury. Above anything else, a design scheme was needed that would bring cohesion not only to San Michele's new extension, but also to the existing parts of the island. Chipperfield's layout created a very strong but flexible framework. Furthermore, the scheme questioned entirely the current cemetery's disposition with nature – with the surrounding water and the sky. The winning proposal rested on a very simple but perceptive observation: that the island's interior fails to live up to its distant poetic view. From afar, the cemetery's high walls seem to suggest a secret garden, or concealed paradise, not unlike those that lie behind dilapidated palazzo walls in Venice itself. In contrast, the landscaping on San Michele errs on the side of mundane. Separated into burial fields or *campi* by red-brick walls similar to those that surround it, it is predominantly given over to roughly mown grass punctuated with indiscriminately placed shrubs, trees and dense rows of graves, crossed with paths. To the north, a large area is laid out as an oppressively rigid labyrinth of modern wall tombs, with row upon row of new funeral marble blocks; walk up the wrong corridor of tombs and you find yourself in a cemetery cul-de-sac, unable to glimpse a way out. You could be anywhere – at least in any other municipal cemetery in Italy. Even the enclosing walls screen the cemetery off from views of the lagoon, and its uniquely beautiful setting. Chipperfield's design for San Michele sets out to restore the discrepancy between appearance and reality – as suggested by its distant view –

through the creation of a real garden for the island.

The garden is to be made out of both enclosed and open spaces. The first stage of the cemetery's extension, which is to be built on an existing *sacca* to the northeast of the present island, is characterised by 'gardens' or physical spaces that are defined largely through tectonic volumes. As external squares and internal courtyards, these spaces have an urban quality. The two main external squares are framed by the exterior walls of the single-storey internal courtyard blocks and the independent set pieces of the scheme – the chapel and the crematorium – whose designs remain unfinalised at the time of writing. The frames of the internal courtyards are formed out of wall tombs. They are colonnaded, making them pleasant places in which to walk or sit. Intentionally more intimate private spaces than the main squares, they are grouped together in blocks of three or four. All the courts differ slightly in size and function, and together form a distinct sequence of spaces. Moreover, each court is to have its own discernible qualities, and thus identity. So, as Chipperfield suggests, you might know the courtyard where your mother is buried by its lemon trees and copper door.[4] This creates a sense of orientation, but moreover of place and belonging.

It is in the second phase of the scheme that the open, garden-like spaces will be established. Constructed on a new strip of land along the eastern edge of the existing island, they will be separated physically from San Michele by a small canal or *rio*. More obviously pastoral in character than the first phase of courtyard spaces – with more area given over to grass – they will visibly set out to readdress the shortcomings of the old cemetery. The architects refer to them directly in their report for the preliminary project as a 'critique of the main island', as they seek to create the 'relationships between walls, gardens, water and views which are conspicuously absent in the existing cemetery'.[5] By creating gardens both outside and within the enclosing wall of the burial grounds, the problem of screening with secure walls – a legal requirement for cemeteries – is overcome. The park-like lower gardens, outside the walls, step down to the water and band the upper gardens that lie within the enclosure. Thus, the lower gardens act as an important transitional space between the island's interior and the lagoon, affording views both of San Michele and its watery setting.

It is only through the construction of higher-density tomb buildings in the northern part of the new island that such a large proportion of open space can be afforded – both with and without burial grounds. For in addition to the estimated 8,941 tombs of the first phase, a further 16,040 are to be provided in the second phase.[6] Though these tomb buildings will be three storeys, rather than the single-storey structures of the

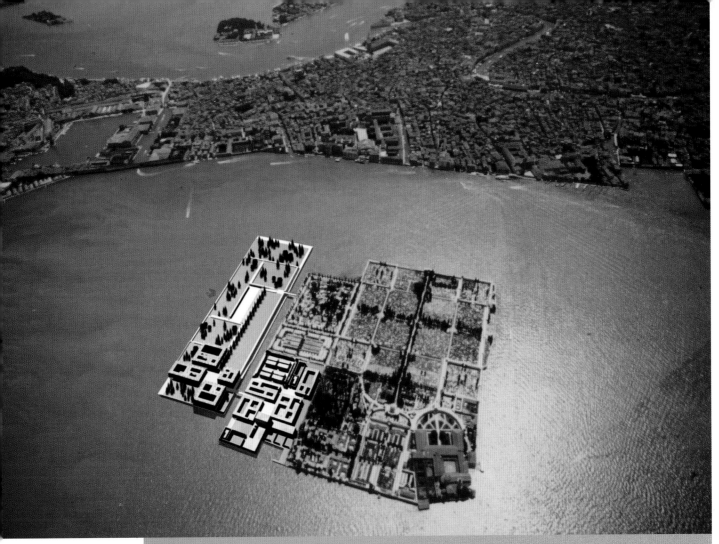

Above
This photomontage of the present island of San Michele with Chipperfield's two planned phases of development pasted on shows its relationship to Venice. The city, which is to the south of the island, here appears above it.

Right
Plan of San Michele. To the northwest is the church of San Michele and the landing stage for the vaporetti. In the north can be seen row upon row of modern wall tombs. To the south are the areas of *campi* separated by high, red-brick walls. Both of Chipperfield's extensions create a striking contrast in their layout to existing areas of the cemetery, which have been driven over the years more by the pressure on space than by design. To the northeast is phase one, with its single-storey courtyard blocks adopting the Venetian urban forms of *calle, campo* and *cortile*. This form is continued to the east in the northern part of the second phase of Chipperfield's design, which forms a separate island, divided from San Michele by a new canal. Here can be seen the expansive areas of open, garden-like space, with areas to the north and the south outside the enclosing cemetery walls, which step down to the lagoon.

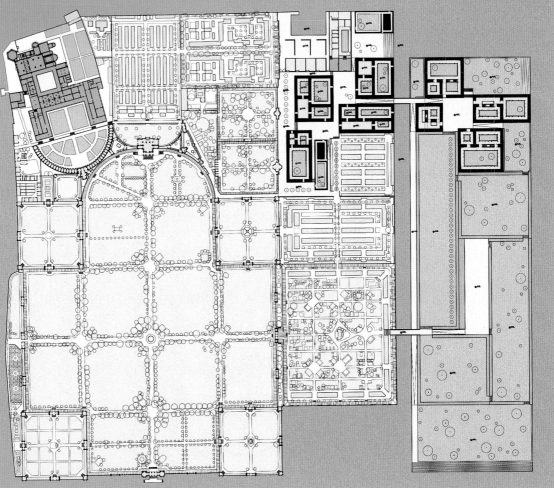

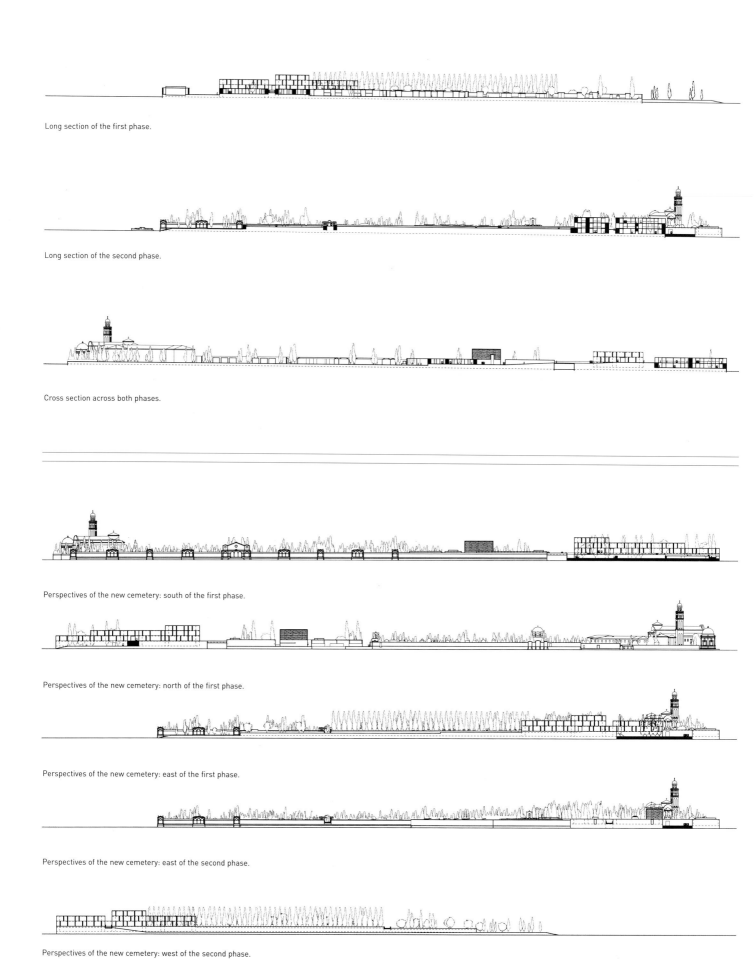

Long section of the first phase.

Long section of the second phase.

Cross section across both phases.

Perspectives of the new cemetery: south of the first phase.

Perspectives of the new cemetery: north of the first phase.

Perspectives of the new cemetery: east of the first phase.

Perspectives of the new cemetery: east of the second phase.

Perspectives of the new cemetery: west of the second phase.

first phase, the two types of building are designed to relate physically and visually. Linked by a bridge, they will adopt a similar use of materials (currently planned as a concrete mix that combines a stone like the traditional *pietra d'Istria*) and similar simple architectural forms. Most importantly, these buildings combine to create a contiguous and seamless settlement that reinterprets the urban pattern of *calle*, *campo* and *cortile* that is so specific to Venice. Thus by imitating the space between buildings rather than the language of the architecture itself, a skilful interpretation of the essential urban qualities of Venice is captured at San Michele. That same experience of abruptly emerging out of the dark of a corridor-like *calle* into the sharp golden light of a *campo*, or entering the cool enclosure of a palazzo's *cortile*, will be encountered in the new cemetery.

Chipperfield's evocation through his built forms of the sensory qualities of Venice reveals a deep recognition of the desire of Venetians to be buried at San Michele. It responds to that strong sense of belonging that the people of Venice already have for their 'island of the dead'. The abstraction of the city's sensory experiences through the contrast of light and shade should be like seeing Venice through half-closed eyes. It is a design tactic that relies on ingenious imitation or interpretation, in the classical sense, rather than historical parody or pastiche. Thus a place related to the city will be created which, at the same time, will stand distinctly apart. The establishment of the garden on the new island will make it less municipal and more park-like than the existing cemetery. So that from the Fondamenta Nuove Venice's final resting place will offer the prospect of a beautiful, irresistible piece of green.

There can be little doubt that the unique geographical and historical position of San Michele colludes towards its ability to procure an architecture of closure at a time when restitution and reconciliation are often conspicuously absent. The relationship between the city and the cemetery is one established through historical continuum rather than contemporary circumstances alone. This in many ways makes it an uneasy paradigm for the 21st century. There is no denying that it does not have to wrangle with the enormity of modern human themes such as the Holocaust, described elsewhere. What it does do, however, is suggest that the possibility of closure – the 'mortal coil' being the most eternal of human themes – might still be sought with sensitivity under the right cultural conditions. ⌂

Notes
1. See p 39.
2. Giulio Lorenzetti, *Venice and its Lagoon: Historical-Artistic Guide*, Edizioni Lint (Trieste), 1975 (reprinted 1985), p 357.
3. The November/December 2000 issue of *Architectural Design* – Fashion and Architecture – will feature an interview with David Chipperfield.
4. From my interview with David Chipperfield, 15 May 2000.
5. 'Ampliamento del Cimitero di San Michele in Isola Veneze', progetto preliminare generale, 10 May 1999, David Chipperfield Architects in collaboration with Jane Wernick Associates, *Ragioni Progettuali*, p 20.
6. Ibid, 1 *Descrizione dei lavori da realizzare*, pp 2–3.

Main sources
Interview 4 May 2000 with Giuseppe Zampieri, project architect at David Chipperfield Architects, and interview 15 May 2000 with David Chipperfield; and 'Ampliamento del Cimitero di San Michele in Isola Veneze', progetto preliminare generale, 10 May 1999, David Chipperfield Architects in collaboration with Jane Wernick Associates.

This page
Original sketches for the San Michele Cemetery.

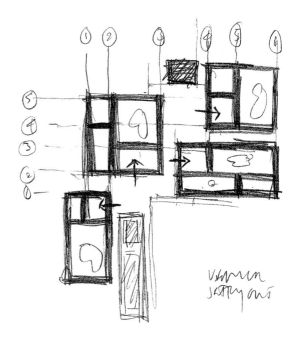

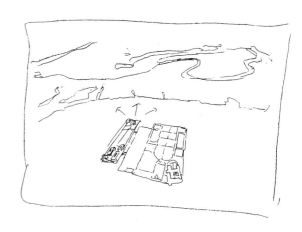

... the fact is that in spite of all the horrors, from Gulag to Holocaust, from capitalism onwards there are no longer tragedies proper – the victims in concentration camps or the victims of the Stalinist show trials were not in a properly tragic predicament; their situation was not without comic – or, at least, ridiculous – aspects; and, for that reason, all the more horrifying – there is a horror so deep that it can no longer be 'sublimated' into tragic dignity, and is for that reason approachable only through an eerie parodic imitation/doubling of the parody itself.

Slavoj Žižek *The Fragile Absolute*

Introduction to the
Holocaust Section

Tragedy is not a concern of the ordinary man, who knows only fear and that sympathy that arises before the spectacle of misfortune. Neither can it be a mere effect of hubris, since hubris is that blindness of pride that may be avoided or corrected by withdrawal into self-reflection and criticism. As the mechanical, inevitable result of actions based on error and illusion, tragedy has no respite and knows only its *telos*. But as Paul Ricoeur noted, it also requires that 'the theme of a predestination to evil of a wicked god come up against the theme of *heroic* greatness'.[1] Plaything of a malignancy, the heroic mortal must suffer not just punishment, but enact catharsis, the purgation of false consciousness or, to use Lacan's words, the dissipation of the 'order' of the imaginary.[2] Cathartic purgation in tragedy, moreover, is said to occur as an effect of language, through the 'sublimity of the poetic word'.[3] Antigone's position, for example, arose from an action based on a criterion of nomination – that of 'brother' – the function of which was to decontextualise her, remove her to an 'eternal' world, away from the historical world of her brother's sin. For Lacan, the poignancy of Antigone's conundrum lay in its reference to a metaphoric shift of 'register', a shift from the characteristics of the historical drama through which one has lived, to 'that purity, that separation of being ... which constitutes 'the life of man'.[4]

The tragic, as genre, serves as a model of social inclusion and responsibility, of the 'proper', in the sense that through it the ordinary man, in becoming a member of the chorus, leaves his pathetic, self-obsessed illusions and enters 'a sphere of feelings that may be called symbolic and mythic'.[5] 'By entering into the tragic "chorus" ourselves, we pass from the Dionysiac illusion to the specific ecstasy of tragic wisdom.'[6] In the modern world, however, our break with illusion, with the drama of historical events, and from the infinity of metonymic inference, can no longer be said to be initiated by self-willed, principled alienation and withdrawal through reflection on the tragic. The fulcrum of our discourse now, in contrast, is the very inaccessibility of the eternal; now it is the very exclusion by which the continuity of historical events might be maintained. This foreclosure of metaphor, the 'Event/Cut', as Žižek calls it, which is 'accessible within time only through its multiple traces',[7] is, of course, the traumatic sublime. It is no longer the symbolic-mythic that anchors social cohesion, but the traumatic. Charles Sargeant Jagger's use of Christ's pose in the crucifixion for his 'ordinary' soldier on the Royal Artillery Memorial at Hyde Park Corner in London (1921–5) is no longer a possible, metaphoric figure of remembrance. Maya Lin poignantly withheld metaphoric signification in the solemn recitation of names for her memorial to Vietnam veterans in Washington DC (1982). In this new order of discourse, it is shared or imagined trauma that must be memorialised and eternalised. It is an unspeakable nature in events that now binds us together as victims, and as such, it is only forms of nomination and location that may be used to inscribe our anxieties. The pre-eminent building type of this new mode of being is the Holocaust memorial. Δ
Richard Patterson

Notes
1. Paul Ricoeur *The Symbolism of Evil*, Harper & Row (New York, Evanston and London), 1967, p 218.
2. Jacques Lacan, *The Ethics of Psychoanalysis 1959–60, The Seminar of Jacques Lacan*, Tavistock/Routledge (London), 1992, p 247.
3. Ricoeur, op cit, p 231.
4. Lacan, op cit, p 279.
5. Ricoeur, op cit, p 222.
6. Ibid, p 231
7. Slavoj Žižek, *The Fragile Absolute*, Verso (London and New York), 2000, p 96.

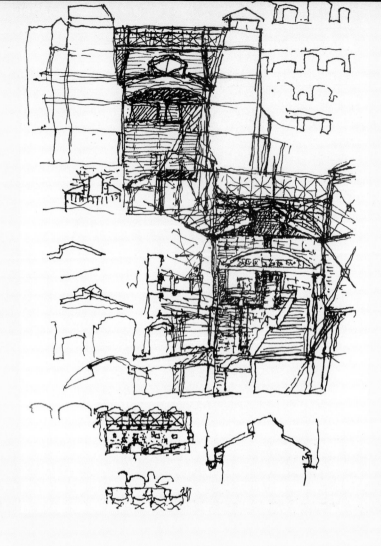

Mapping Tragedy
in the US Holocaust
Memorial Museum

The extraordinary significance of the Holocaust for the United States belies the fact of its geographic distance from the original events. Thus aesthetic constructs commemorating the Holocaust in the US, situated out of context and sometimes in overdetermined locations, may act more as records of destruction than as memorials. How then, does a monument stimulate rather than obliterate memory, and what type of architecture is appropriate for such a building? Joan Branham explores how James Ingo Freed has addressed these questions through the structure of tragic narrative in his US Holocaust Memorial Museum in Washington DC.

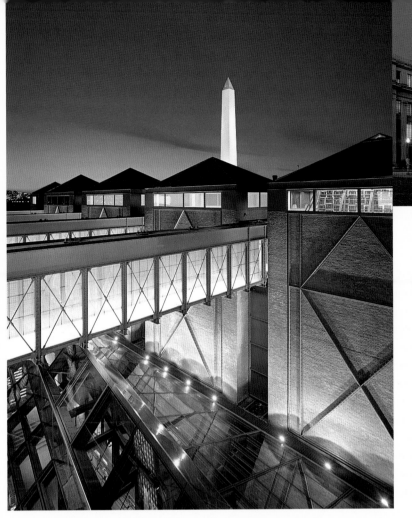

Designing the Holocaust

Some would argue that the term 'Holocaust art' is an oxymoron consisting of two mutually contradictory signifiers – one indicating all that is base, evil and blind in the human experience, the other designating everything transcendent, worthy and visionary in the human spirit. How can the Holocaust, an event that pushes the very limits of describability and comprehension, be represented in aesthetic terms? Is it possible to translate tragedy and atrocity into paint on canvas, poetry on paper, musical notes or architectural design? Perhaps even more enigmatic is the Holocaust's ironic ability to engender art. At the centre of these perplexities stands James Ingo Freed's architectural overture, the US Holocaust Memorial Museum in Washington DC.

Since its commission and supervision by the US Holocaust Memorial Council in 1980, the project has been fraught with controversy. First, the site of the building in the nation's capital – adjacent to the Mall and part of the sacred American landscape – has elicited ambivalence and anxiety from several quarters. To design and construct what some have dubbed 'a national Jewish cathedral'[1] alongside the Jefferson Memorial and Washington Monument thrusts Jewish presence and identity into the American public's awareness, but solely in terms of the Holocaust, that is to say, the destruction of Judaism.[2]

Memorials, by their very nature, pose other dangers. James Young has written at length on the tendency of individuals to displace their own 'memory work' on to externalised, static monuments which ironically, but intrinsically, end up usurping the individual's mandate to remember instead of provoking it.[3] How then does a monumental space of immense proportions, situated in a charged and overdetermined location, negotiate the fine line between soliciting and supplanting memory?

And finally, from a design perspective, the memorial museum gives rise to a number of conceptual challenges. A beautiful building would risk adorning the Holocaust and thus rendering it palatable. A literal design, recapitulating the architecture of Nazi camps, would trivialise the Holocaust by creating a simulacrum. And a completely neutral structure, designed to frame but not engage its internal collection, would admit the inability of contemporary architecture to exercise form as a mechanism of meaning and responsibility. In the words of architectural critic Paul Goldberger, the task was 'inherently impossible' from the outset.[4]

In 1986, the Nobel Peace Prize-winning writer Elie Wiesel announced the appointment of James Ingo Freed (presently of Pei, Cobb, Freed & Partners) as the architect to confront these seemingly insurmountable challenges. Responding to ambivalence around the museum project, Wiesel stated, 'the Holocaust in its enormity defies language and art, and yet both must be used to tell the tale, the tale that must be told'.[5] Freed's resulting architectural design manifests the literary underpinnings of Wiesel's use of the term 'tale', for the US Holocaust Memorial Museum is a building based on narrative structure and in turn cognisant of the narrative-driven collection it accommodates. If nothing else, Freed's museum design may be one of the 20th century's most successful examples of architectural form in dialogue with its very contents, an external shell intimately connected to and dictated by internal matter. Of interest to us here, then, is the relationship between architectural composition, exhibition substance and the narrative genre of tragedy.

Space as Narrative

Mapped out along a sequential topography, the museum's exhibition begins on the fourth floor and works in chronological progression and spatial descent. The visitor follows the primary narrative plot from Hitler's rise to power on the third floor, to internment in camps and ghettos on the second floor, and finally to liberation on the first floor. Along the narrative journey,

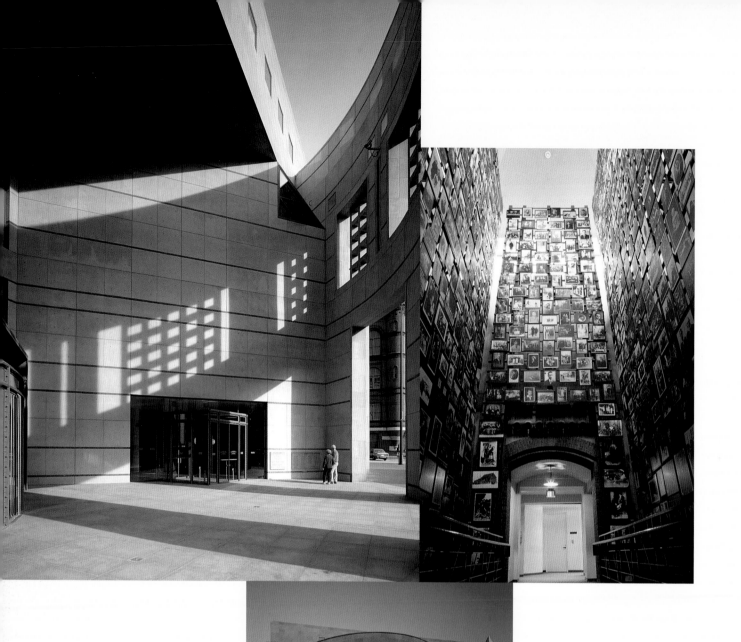

Top left
Inside the 'screen' to the 14th Street entrance.

Top right
The Tower of Faces.

Middle
14th Street facade.

Bottom
View of Hall of Witnesses.

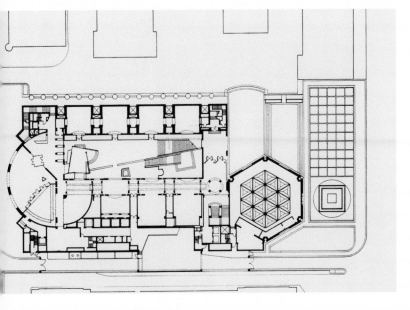

the exhibition materials introduce the visitor to the leading characters in the story: protagonists, perpetrators, victims, bystanders, rescuers and liberators.[6] In fact, the narrative journey begins with a feature similar to the literary genre of tragedy: the audience's identification with a protagonist. Upon entering the museum's space, we are given a passport with the name, picture and story of a real Holocaust victim. The viewer not only reads about and empathises with such protagonists, but actually encounters them along the way through synecdochal remnants such as hair, shoes, suitcases and wedding rings. These relics are genuine, of course, and move this narrative space beyond the literary limits of representation into the realm of the corporeal, tangible and real. Tragic narrative merges with palpable environment.

The Tower of Faces, possibly the most potent narrative space in the museum, realises a seamless rapport between architectural design and material collection. Here, Freed punctuates the larger architectural narrative of the museum with a three-storey tower housing 1,500 photographs of inhabitants from the Polish *shtetl* Ejszyski. A sub narrative emerges of the massacre of 4,000 Jews in a single village by Nazi mobile killing squads on Rosh Hashanah in 1941. Within two days, the entire Jewish population of this village was obliterated. We learn that one survivor – yet another internal narrative – Yaffa Sonenson Eliach has spent the rest of her life collecting photographs of people from her village before it was wiped out.[7] What we see, then, are pre-Nazi images of life, not death – of children dressed up for their school pictures, young girls posing dramatically à la

Hollywood, couples taking their marriage vows, and families on holiday. Freed does not merely line the walls of the tower with these compelling images, but uses the photographs as a building material to construct the tower's very walls. In so doing, he undermines the traditional role of the museum as 'container for images' and merges exhibition materials and museum space into one integrated and interdependent construct.

In the Tower of Faces, Freed further reverses the architectural iconography of the watchtower – a structure normally associated with the close monitoring of victims and their movements – by creating an introspective edifice where gaze and scrutiny take place on the inside. The victims, bathed in natural sunlight from above, look out at us as we pass through their space on a semi transparent, 7 foot bridge. The visitor, the bridge, the photographs and the actual lives of the victims are all simultaneously and symbolically suspended in this multivalent space, where compound layers of narrative unfold before our eyes.

Mimetic Subversions

Freed's appropriation and reinterpretation of Holocaust forms such as the watchtower describe the governing design principle for the rest of the museum. Freed states, 'I was not interested in resuscitating the forms of the Holocaust'.[8] Instead, he alludes to Holocaust forms in a deliberate, unapologetic, but critical manner. For example, the Hall of Remembrance, a hexagonal structure attached to the main building, is a metaphor for the six sides of the yellow star that Jews were forced to wear, as well as the six million who were murdered. The external walls of this hall do not actually meet each other to create a unified structure, but fall short of closure. In Freed's own words, 'we wanted an evocation of the incomplete. Irresolution, imbalances are built in'.[9] In the Hall of Remembrance, any attempt to finalise or determine memory collapses.

The 14th Street entrance to the museum discloses another emergent Holocaust motif. Here, the visitor encounters a false entrance, a deceptive screen that announces 'threshold' in a monumental way. Two huge pillars symmetrically separate three entry portals, recalling the posturing of Neoclassical forms. Upon penetrating the screen, however, the viewer realises that the portico gives way only to a shallow courtyard open to the sky; one must move off axis to seek an alternative entrance. Freed remarks:

The concentration camps all had gates, layers of lies, lies such as *Arbeit macht frei* (work makes free). The gate as lie, screen ... a pure façade, a pure fake ... You pass through the limestone screen to enter a concrete world. We disorient you, shifting and re-centring you three times, to separate you emotionally as well as visually from Washington.[10]

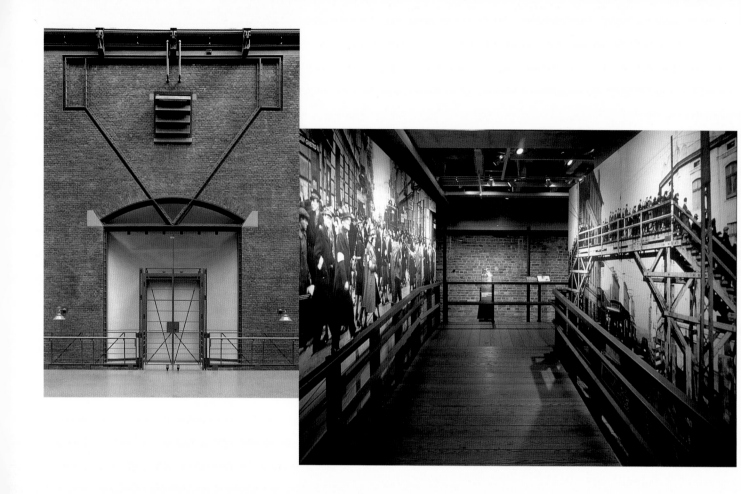

'We always deal in dualities: dark and light, transparency and opacity. Everywhere there are two options: down or up, left or right.'

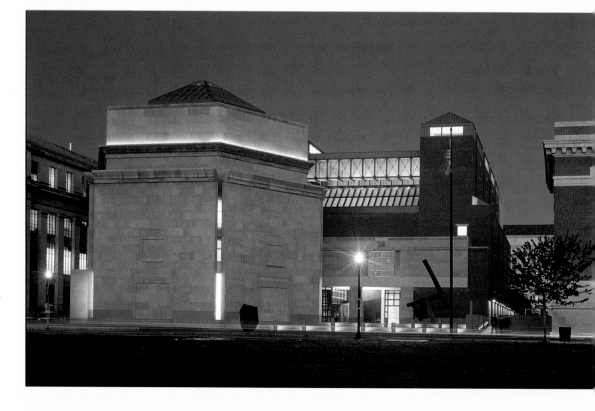

Above left
Architectural detail of brick and metal above doorway.

Above right
Ghetto footbridge with murals of Jews taking bridges above non-Jewish streets.

Bottom
15th Street Facade

Opposite
Hall of Witnesses

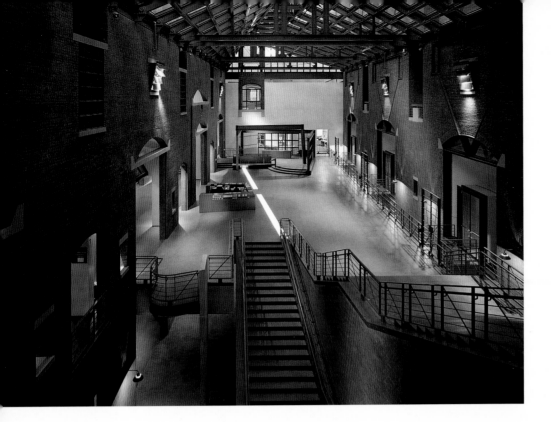

Notes
1. See Peter Novick's discussion in *The Holocaust in American Life*, Houghton Mifflin Company (Boston), 1999, p 199, as well as Eva Hoffman's insightful review of his book in 'The Uses of Hell', *The New York Review of Books*, 9 March 2000, pp 19–23.
2. For a more expanded discussion of this and other museums as sacred landscapes, see my article, 'Sacrality and Aura in the Museum: Mute Objects and Articulate Space', *The Journal of the Walters Art Gallery*, vol 52/53, 1994/95, pp 33–47.
3. Young specifically deals with this issue in a fascinating chapter, 'The Countermonument: Memory Against Itself in Germany', *The Texture of Memory*, Yale University Press (New Haven), 1993, pp 27–48.
4. Paul Goldberger, 'A Memorial Evokes Unspeakable Events with Dignity', *New York Times*, 30 April 1989.
5. Herbert Muschamp, 'Shaping a Monument to Memory', *New York Times*, 11 April 1993, Section 2.
6. See Jeshajahu Weinberg and Rina Elieli, *The Holocaust Museum in Washington*, Rizzoli (New York), 1995, pp 17, 49.
7. See Susan Brenna, 'Images of a Vanished Town', *New York Newsday*, 17 March 1991.
8. From an interview with Freed in 'James Ingo Freed: The United States Holocaust Memorial Museum', *Assemblage 9*, 1989, p 65.
9. Ibid p 64.
10. Ibid, pp 62, 65.
11. Ibid, p 70.
12. Ibid, p 62.
13. See Adrian Dannatt, *United States Holocaust Memorial Museum: James Ingo Freed*, Phaidon Press (London), 1995, pp 6–7.
14. Freed, pp 63–4.
15. Ibid, p 65.

In contradistinction to other Washington monuments, whose primary purpose is to draw you into the Washington landscape, the US Holocaust Memorial Museum distances the visitor from the authoritative language of democracy and patriotism in preparation to meet the Shoah.

Freed's symbolic incorporation of Holocaust motifs is not limited to the optical panorama alone, but materialises in the visitor's spatial experience as well. Freed choreographs the participant's movement through the museum's space, forcing the guest to make narrative choices. At the entrance, visitors must discriminate between two doors: one for groups, one for individuals. Freed explains: 'We made the two entries different. Visitors will experience a selection, a segregation of movement, arbitrary ... We always deal in dualities: dark and light, transparency and opacity. Everywhere there are two options: down or up, left or right.'[11]

This ability to manipulate the trajectories of visitors in the museum proves to be one of Freed's strengths. His previous design experience, most notably with the Jacob K Javits Convention Center in New York, gave him incomparable training in moving large masses of people. In the Holocaust museum, however, crowd control becomes more than a logistical issue: it conjures a tragic narrative in itself, weighty with symbolism. Referring to Nazi-based systems of crowd control, Freed notes that victims first experienced 'alienation, separation from the body politic. Then there's transportation, then concentration. Then there is death'.[12] Freed himself is no stranger to movement and relocation, having experienced the transportative element of the Holocaust first-hand as a boy. Born in Essen, Germany, in 1930, he was moved, along with his sister, from Germany to France, from France to Switzerland, and finally from Europe to Chicago in order to avoid the ever-pursuing Nazis.[13] Consequently, path, pattern and map figure prominently in his design. His use of footbridges, for example, to transport the public from one space to another in the museum, are reminiscent of the wooden footbridges constructed by the Nazis to carry Jewish pedestrians over 'non-Jewish streets' in the Warsaw ghetto.

Ultimately, Freed's most unmitigated appropriation, subversion and reinvention of Holocaust forms derive from the brick ovens of camp crematoria. He remarks: 'If you look at the ovens at Auschwitz, you can see that they are strapped together with steel. Originally they were built out of brick, but the steel strapping was needed because the ovens were so overused that they tended to explode from internal gases ... The addition of heavy steel to a raw wall became for me a very important thing.'[14]

Indeed, the museum's interior and exterior are in large part composed of brickwork riveted with metal bands. Freed's architectural application of Holocaust forms is, however, far from literal or imitative. Here, as in the Tower of Faces, he transforms the iconography of destruction into construction, the risks and hazards of the project into its strengths. Instead of simulating the real, the museum converses with the genuine objects it encloses, be they authentic barracks from Auschwitz, a cattle car used to transport Jews, or Nazi uniforms. In the US Holocaust Memorial Museum Freed has responded to tragedy by embracing and translating narrative structure into architectural form to tell the tale that must be told, and in Freed's own words, to summon forth 'visceral memory, visceral as well as visual'.[15] ◬

whole spectrum of German political identity since the Second World War. At the moment of Germany's reunification, in the spirit of hope for the future, it seemed appropriate that the new German state should somehow lay to rest the ghosts of past regimes. This has taken many forms, including a symbolic register of the horrors of the Holocaust – a proposed memorial sited in the vicinity of the new government buildings in Berlin. Astrid Schmeing traces the many layers of inference and interpretation that coloured its reception.

After the war, the Allies mounted posters in Germany's cities featuring a photograph of a scene in a concentration camp. These were part of the Allies' re-education programme, which aimed to teach a whole population to become 'good democrats'. Each was headed with the words 'You Are Guilty', an admonition addressed to every German individual. They were directed towards a society that had identified discipline, strength, obedience and a strong belief in authority as its core virtues; a society that supported its *Führer* even towards the end of the war. The words 'You Are Guilty' demand the rational individual sense of responsibility that forms the basis of modern, democratic society.

Within the context of modernism, the Holocaust cannot be grasped and, yet, cannot be forgotten. How could it have happened in a

surrounded by busy streets, in the centre of Berlin. On three sides are foreign embassies and housing, with the fourth side, to the west, facing the Tiergarten, Berlin's largest park. It is located near the Reichstag, the Brandenburg Gate and Potsdamer Platz, all of which can be seen from the site. In 1999, the decision was taken to construct the memorial according to a design by Peter Eisenman. This design had been reworked from an earlier, competition-winning version submitted by Eisenman and Richard Serra (see overleaf).[2] The original proposal by Eisenman/Serra presented itself as 'minimalist': a moving topography of more than 4,000 pillars, rising from 'zero' at ground level to a height of 7 metres. Each of the pillars was to be 230 x 92 centimetres in plan, set 92 centimetres apart in a slightly angled, irregular manner. The memorial was to fill the whole of the block, up to the boundary with the streets. The only possible way of experiencing it would

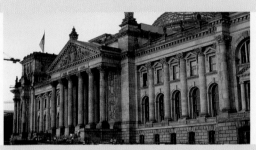

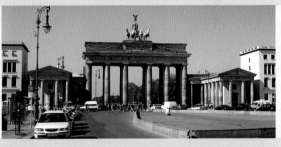

civilised country and how can we ensure that nothing like it ever happens again? The Holocaust is not simply a historical detail that can be left behind as an enduring possibility that must to be avoided, however. It is a matter of the human condition, rather than a national, German issue. Nevertheless, within the context of affiliated European nation states, and a unified German nation, it remains a German question. And, especially with German reunification, the question of what 'nation' means has become pre-eminent. Can the term still be used in a traditional sense? Helmut Kohl, the German chancellor from 1982 to 1999, certainly used it as such. He defined 'nation' not only as a linguistic, territorial and legal community, but as one identified by common tradition, religion and culture.[1] That is to say, he defined it in an irrational, determinist and fatalistic way, which contradicts the rational-individual position sketched out above.

For the past 12 years, a proposed memorial for the murdered Jews of Europe has acted as a catalyst for a wide-ranging debate concerning the way in which Germans relate to the Nazi past and the Holocaust and, in consequence, how they define themselves as a nation. A site was designated, which fills a whole 'block', entirely

therefore have been as an 'individual', since no two people could have moved next to each other in these narrow spaces.

The field of pillars in this proposal appears at first glance to be inaccessible, incomprehensible. What is the relationship between this minimalist site and the memory of Europe's Jews and how they were murdered? An interesting answer perhaps lies in its very minimalism, which has been discussed with reference to sculpture by Rosalind Krauss:

In their seemingly obdurate refusal to transform the commonplace, the minimalist sculptors produced work that appeared to be aspiring toward the condition of non-art, to be breaking down any distinction between the world of art and the world of everyday objects. What their work seemed to share with those objects was a fundamental property that went deeper than the mere fact of banality of the materials used. That property one might describe as the inarticulate existence of the object. The way the object seems merely to perpetuate itself in space and time in terms of the repeated occasions of its use. So that we might say of a chair or table, that beyond knowing its function, one has no other way to get the 'meaning' out of it.[3]

The memorial's minimalist abstraction refuses to provide a meaning beyond its name: Memorial for the Murdered Jews of Europe. Like minimalism in

There is no figure, and one does not even face an 'object'. Instead, the individual moves within and inside the components of the memorial.

sculpture, the memorial aspires towards the condition of non-art: it becomes 'real'. It is not a representation of memory so much as it is part of memory. It is an unconventional memorial that does not suggest how to remember. A conventional memorial would perhaps provide a figure to be 'looked at'. The figurative object, witnessed by the observer's external perspective, would provide a sense of wholeness or 'completion', which would suggest 'how to remember'. This memorial, however, refuses to do so. There is no figure, and one does not even face an 'object'. Instead, the individual moves within and inside the components of the memorial. One's body becomes involved as a part of it, and the memorial is only complete when faced by each, single participating observer. Any form of memory transported to it by the observer becomes part of the memorial.

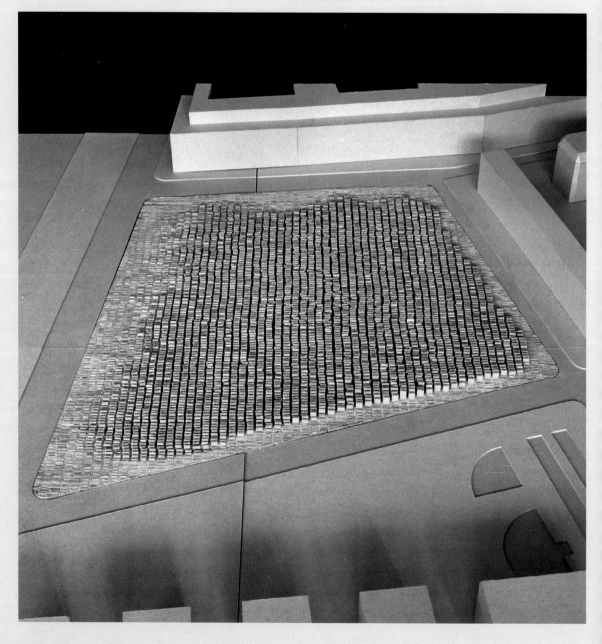

Model of the original competition-winning proposal for the memorial designed by Peter Eisenman and Richard Serra.

Integrating different individuals and therefore different possibilities of completion and interpretation, the memorial can be claimed to be a democratic one. Jürgen Habermas writes:

In late modernism there is no commonly shared context left in which traditional, symbolic expressions and ritualised practices can produce collective bindings without reason. Today, the effect of a memorial that does not aesthetically fail always sustains the varying reservoir of reasons that conditioned its construction. On the other hand, a nation's cultural memory, which should not be confused with private memory, cannot solely be reproduced in the discursive medium of history writing, literature and teaching.[4]

According to Habermas, in a modern democracy the individual is not relieved of a critical attitude towards the mechanisms of his or her own behaviour. With regards to commemorating the Holocaust, this means that it is neither possible to relate uncritically to one's own cultural context, nor to distance oneself uncritically. With this unconventional memorial, the design refers to the modernist context that Habermas has sketched out, though one might doubt whether it is really able to enforce an individual and critical position, or whether it simply allows the individual, but non reflected, memory to be projected on to it. Whatever may be the case, this non representative design does not invite collective bonding in the way that a figurative object would do.

For the greater part of the competition assessment a conservative government was in power, headed by Helmut Kohl. When the German parliament came to decide the winning entry he interfered directly in the process, indicating his preference for the Eisenman/Serra entry. One might ask why Kohl, a conservative, favoured this unconventional memorial which, as we have argued, invited individual responsibility and seemingly precluded the possibility of the kind of national identification that might be promulgated by his party. To find the answer, one needs to examine what happened next. Kohl asked Eisenman and Serra to rework their scheme, causing Serra to drop out. Kohl's suggested changes, far from superficial, fundamentally transformed the meaning of the memorial, introducing elements of communal experience and civic ritual.

In the original plan, the memorial extended to the edges of the site; pedestrians who wanted to avoid it or pass it by would have to have crossed to the other side of the street, again creating a situation whereby the only possible experience of the memorial would have been

The memorial has become an object that can be perceived from the outside, returning to the notion of a conventional memorial that asks for irrational identification.

an individual one. Kohl asked Eisenman to reduce the number and height of pillars, so that they would become less dominant, to integrate trees, a space for buses to park and, most importantly, a designated place for the laying of wreaths. As a result, the urban block would no longer determine the memorial's size. It would allow pedestrians to stroll along its edges and perceive it as an object from the outside. What the pedestrians would see – the field of pillars – would not be as abstract as before, but would allow the figurative analogy of a graveyard to be made. The memorial had become an object that could be perceived from the outside, returning to the notion of a conventional memorial that asks for irrational identification. The motif of a graveyard – although a symbol for mourning, which had always been one of the intentions for the memorial – has different implications. For the graveyard is not only a Jewish symbol; it is also Christian, which fits perfectly with the politics of Kohl and the postwar conservatives.

After the war, the conservatives argued against the principle that every individual had been responsible for the Holocaust ('You Are Guilty'), for the simple reason that a rational, individual approach to responsibility made it difficult to mourn the nation's 'own' dead,

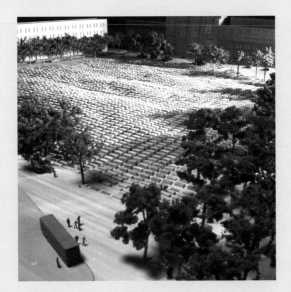

Right
View of the model of the Eisenman 2 memorial scheme, looking from southwest towards the northeast.

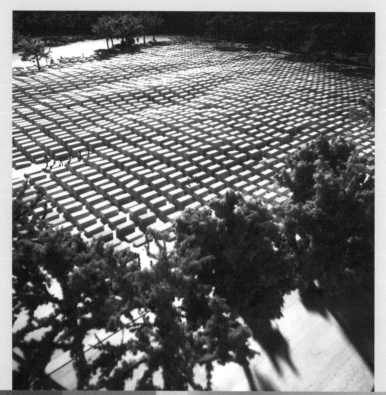

Bottom
Aerial view of a model of the new Eisenman 2 scheme. Here, the site has been reduced to include fewer pillars and to allow for the mandatory pavement and adequate circulation. To the left is the proposed site for the American Embassy; in the middle of the block is a bank building by Frank Gehry, and at the end an art and science building by Oswald Ungers. On the right is a proposed office block.

Right
Model of the new Eisenman 2 memorial scheme, looking from the northeast towards the southwest.

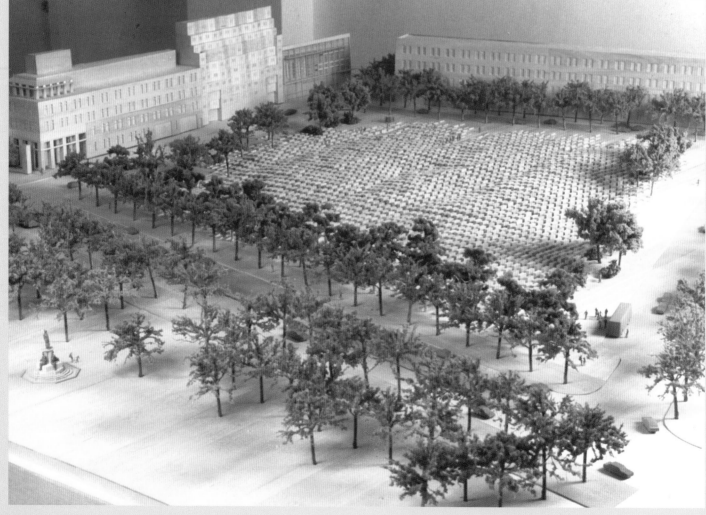

especially the soldiers who had perished on the Eastern Front. They were thought to have given their life for their nation, but at the same time, objectively, they had allowed the continuation of the Holocaust, the Jewish *Todesmärsche* ('march to the death') and the mass murder of the camps. A rational, responsible individual position would not give the space to mourn them uncritically. A Christian position in which the dead are all equal, however, would do just that. The symbol of the graveyard would therefore allow for a universal mourning for all who died.

The conflict between memorialising the soldiers of the Eastern Front and accepting responsibility for the Holocaust is also a problem for national identity, since it does not allow for belief in the virtue of one's 'own' nation. Within the German conservative ideology 'responsibility' is not ascribed to the nation, but to the totalitarian system, to Hitler's dictatorship, allowing 'Germans' to be seen as Hitler's first victims. It is the state that has power and it is the state that exercises responsibility; no critical question remains for the 'nation' to answer. The second phase of the memorial has become, in this sense, a state memorial rather than an individual one, since the message it transmits is fundamentally that of differentiating the democratic Federal Republic from the totalitarian Third Reich. In these terms, the memorial is affirmative: it states the difference between the two systems, and acts as a positive reinforcement for the former. The nation is now attached to a 'good state', which, in return, depends upon national identification for its survival.

In the reworked design, is that the memorial offers itself as a communal event. The observer is no longer isolated amongst the pillars. The space for the laying of wreaths is now assigned as such, created to enable communal/political rituals to take place. This makes the differentiation between Nazi Germany and the FRG even more explicitly manifest.

The modernist reading – that of individual experience and the possibility of an infinite number of different readings – still coexists in this memorial, however. There remains something undecided about it, which allows it to act as a democratic signifier: the possibility now exists for the projection of different sets of values, transforming it over time. Though not necessarily either modern or rational, it still has the potential to be a truly democratic, symbolic memorial. ⌂

Notes
1. Helmut Kohl, 'Zwischen Ideologie und Pragmatismus, Aspekte und Ansichten' zu Grundfragen der Politik, *Bonn Aktuell*, 1973.
2. The reworked 1999 version by Eisenman is now subject to a further revision, to include a new 'didactic' element. Its content and form are not yet determined.
3. Rosalind Krauss, *Passages in Modern Sculpture* MIT (Cambridge), seventh edition, 1989, p 189.
4. Jürgen Habermas, 'Der Zeigefinger. Die Deutschen und 1hr Denkmal', *Die Zeit*, no 14, 31 March 1999: 'In der späten Moderne gibt es keinen allgemein geteilten Kontext mehr, worin überlieferte symbolische Ausdrucksformen und rituelle Praktiken begründungsfrei kollektive Verbindlichkeiten erzeugen könnten. Die Wirkung eines Denkmals, das ästhetisch nicht mißlingt, zehrt heute immer auch vom schwankenden Reservoir der Gründe, die zu seiner Errichtung geführt haben. Andererseits kann sich das kulturelle Gedächtnis einer Nation, das ja nicht mit privater Erinnerung verwechselt werden darf, nicht allein im diskursiven Medium von Geschichtsschreibung, Literatur und Unterricht fortpflanzen.'

The Voic

Libeskind's Jewish Museum, Berlin

hat is Subject

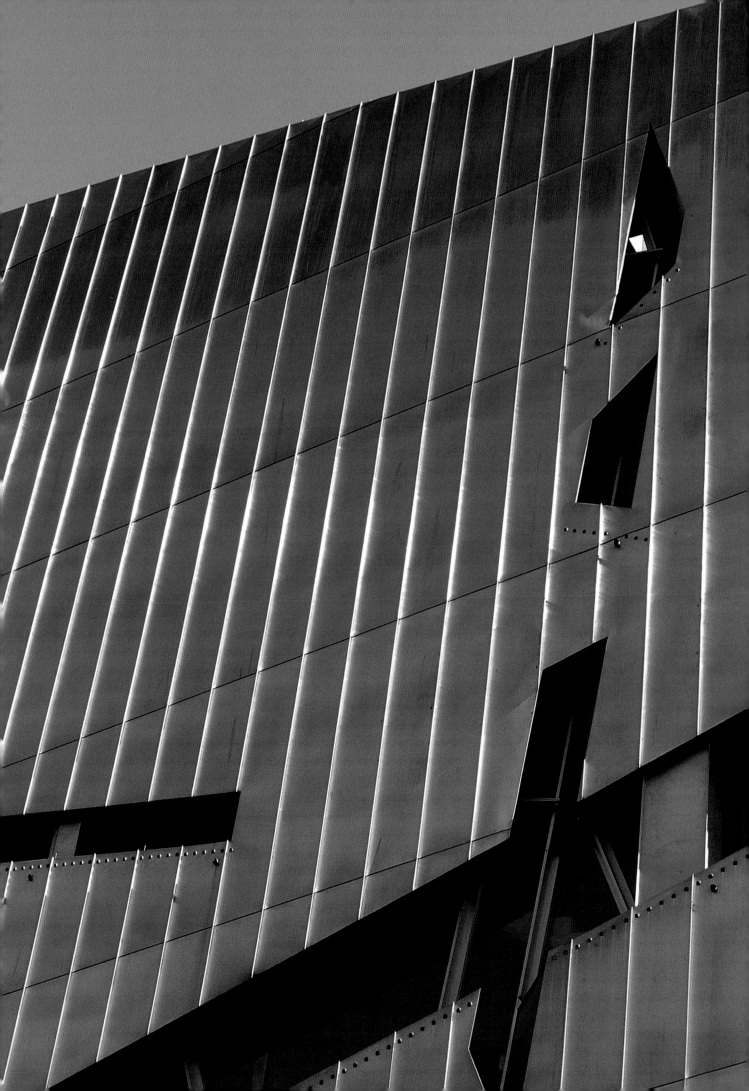

A museum dedicated to the history of the Jews in Berlin cannot be easily circumscribed in programmatic terms. The architecture by which Daniel Libeskind has realised his remarkable Jewish Museum is innovative at the level of communion rather than as architectural performance and display. Richard Patterson examines the formal basis of his achievement.

Berlin lies on the Brandenburg plain, some way from the irregularities of landscape that normally occupy one's attention from the air. Rivers form a skein of waterways that, from a moving perspective, create a silver wave of reflected light travelling across the landscape. Arrival at Tegel airport is low-key, and in September it was very warm. Berlin is perhaps the most modest of European capital cities. Nowhere is this more evident than at Sans Souci, often compared with Versailles but with which it has nothing in common. The palace is a model of aspiration and achievement, its gardens, Weinterrasse, evoking a precise sublimation of their prototype. This imperial residence grips its location self-consciously, rigorously and overtly, yet in so restrained a way as to appear to tell the literal truth about things as they are. In fantasy, Berlin is the city of spies, cabaret, Isherwood; a city of damp, grimy stone infrastructure, of sandbags and guard posts. Or of Karl Friedrich Schinkel. And Schinkel is now all the more evident, since the removal of the wall has enabled the old urban forms to reassert themselves, while the various gestures of modernism, which had seemed to epitomise the postwar period, appear to be lost in their particular historical moments. Within this invisible repair of the historical soul, Daniel Libeskind has inserted a memorial destined to keep the wounds fresh.

The closest U-bahn station to the Jewish Museum is Hallisches Tor, from which one passes through a modern residential district. The architecture of this area is of a high quality, leafy, sunny and replete with a variety of pedestrians and domestic animals. It is in the midst of this hallucination of emphatic normalcy that the museum seems to emerge, framed by trees and the pavement, across the street, glinting in the sunlight, new and silvery, with inexplicable and violent incisions slicing across its skin. Its geometry is not that of its context. A lack of signage signifies that this is not commercial attention-seeking. The visitor in September was still barred from approaching the building by a high, wire construction hoarding, punctuated with barbed wire along its top and vertically in the more awkward conjunctions of its panels. One day, the zinc cladding will mellow to a matt grey, softer and more like the sky, and the museum will fade somewhat into Berlin. There is a garden, and people are tending it. There are railway tracks leading right up to and under the building, but no evident way in.

I walked around the back and then through a small park, in what may have been a garden along the edge of the Collegienhaus (or the Museum of Berlin, which is the entrance to the Jewish Museum), and up to a point at the front, on the Lindenstrasse, where the fence stopped. A benign-looking, West-German-style policeman was standing nearby in the sunlight, across from a small gap through which one might squeeze, past the detritus, up to the front door. A group of tourists in possession of appropriate documentation had appeared and were being granted admission. Absent-mindedly passing through the door, my attention was engaged by a smiling attendant of immaculate politeness: 'Besuchen Sie das Museum?'

Although the museum is not yet officially open (completed in January 1999, it will not be formally opened until approximately 2002), it already has a level of attendance that is second only to the Pergamon Museum, the foremost of German classical collection and location of the Pergamon altar. There are no exhibits yet, but there are guided tours, organised by the Museumspedagogischesdienst, for which printed tickets are sold. During my visit there were around five or six different tours in progress. People come to see the building and hear the story of its creation.

Entrance to the Jewish Museum proper is made by way of a stair that is set at an angle to the geometry of the Collegienhaus. It reminded me of the descent into one of the cellars at Epernay, or perhaps a silver mine in Nevada. There is no colour, but shades of grey. At basement level, the floors slope slightly in various directions through a system of corridors. There is little detail, although there are display cases resembling shop windows, which are built into the walls. This area is a world of street corners, and it is disorienting. This light is artificial as it is night-time. The guide indicates the different directions, and names their various objectives. What everyone is really interested in, however, is the line dividing the 'old' from the 'new' construction, the Collegienhaus from the Jewish Museum. This distinction, it turns out, is signified by a movement joint, which is then inspected carefully by all. They want to know where they are, where they stand. They are actively fighting the disorientation.

The main stair comes as a surprise. The return to natural light is like waking up. At ground level are two cruciform windows from which one can catch sight of the garden, of flowers and colour and more light. The glazing of these openings is flush with the inner face of the wall and this, along with the narrowness of their shape, requires one to peer at the exterior. It is this detail that has created the strong visual impression of incisions on the exterior of the building. On the inside, it produces a sense of isolation and claustrophobia. The stair rises from bottom to top and is, as it were, unending. The light is evocative and full. From the top,

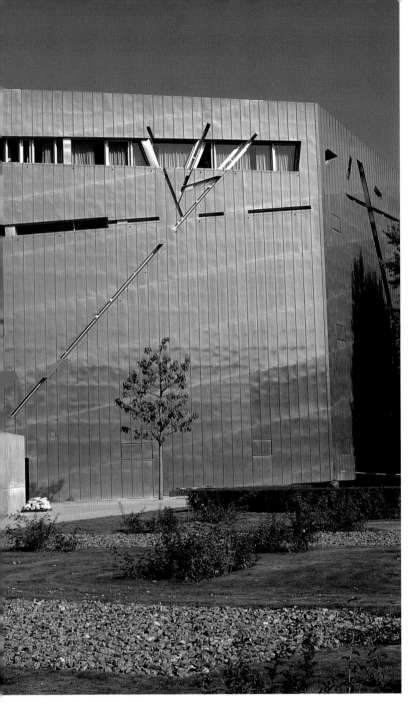

looking back, one notices more fully the concatenation of struts supporting the outer wall. A memory of Libeskind's skill as a draughtsman is evident in such details. They appear to be the result of some arbitrary or transient event, but their form is powerful enough to sustain them, irrespective of their place in the building.

It had occurred to me from studying Libeskind's drawings that the building was very simple. The section is direct, complete and box-like. It is just accommodation for a series of exhibits. It has the glass-to-glass dimension and constancy of height that defines a certain type of modern conception: the rational office building. The interiors of the Jewish Museum are black, white and grey; the floor is terrazzo; the walls and ceiling are emulsion on plaster. The effect is one of unyielding ordinariness, and is entirely different from what I had anticipated, based on

Libeskind's graphic surfaces. The electrostatic energy of those surfaces – as inferred from the visual reverberations of form to be drawn from the dimension lines on the published plans – is simply not evident to the visitor. The plan, which was famously derived from the geometry of the Star of David, meanders discursively, in a manner of speaking, unpredictably, creating, with the intrusion of the vertical cores, a seeming labyrinth of nooks and crannies. The general opinion seems to be that the building is at its most sculpturally powerful now, and that it will be lessened by the exhibits. One imagines from the recently opened Nussbaum Museum, also by Libeskind, that these exhibits will have certain unique qualities, in that they will occasionally be things in the space of the museum, occasionally constructions with their own distinct, internal narratives, occasionally contrived (organised, placed on the wall, assisted by signage, etc) in such a way as to collude with the form of the museum itself. The deconstructive moment of this sublime work, however, will lie in its corrosive impact on these received wisdoms, this narrative, this didactic museological discourse. It will not be that the museum draws our attention away from these objects, but that the mechanism of it will subvert those defensive reifications we so avidly manufacture from the splintered texture of our observations. The dream of the absent-minded aesthetic gaze, the disinterested gaze of the passive witness, will be a disturbed dream as the varying registers of our perception and reflection come to be manipulated in this way. Because this is not a labyrinth; this is one building where you always know where you are.

In our Cartesian model of experience, the subject, the *cogito*, 'I', is 'here', and the object of my perceptions is 'there', in the form of something 'other'. As for 'architecture', I observe or enter a space that I 'understand' insomuch as it is constituted of those abstract and universal principles that are the proper objects of mathematics or psychology, and, as such, are said to be the objective basis of experience and cognition. According to the 'empiricist sequence', I 'suffer sensations that lead to perceptions and then to "ideas".'[1] In both cases, the building I encounter is objectively 'there', and the meanings I read in it are due to its objective situation, context, and formal and historical references – the naturalism of its construction, its function and so on – to the extent that anything that is not 'there', that is nonetheless a part of my experience, must be due to personal fantasy and imagination. Some time ago, Anthony Vidler devised a typological set for classifying the inherent rationality of architecture, which included construction, function, and, something radically new: the linguistic property of formal, architectural paradigms. On this basis, it was intended to ground architecture on its own terms,

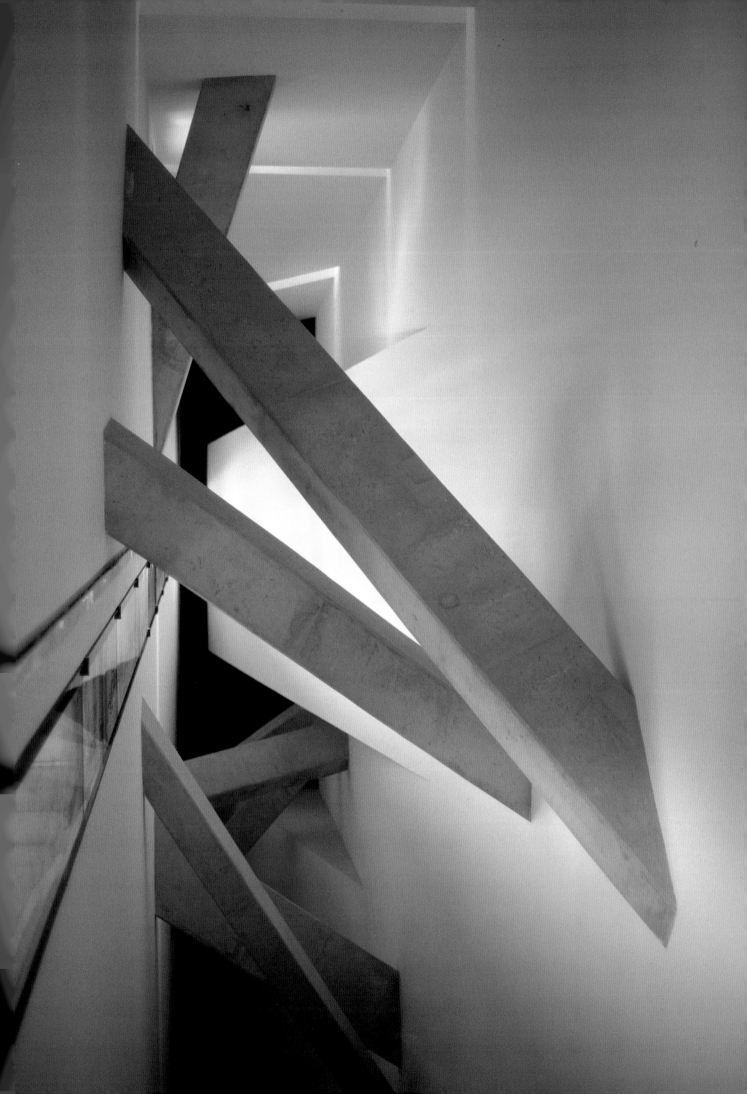

without reference to external demands. At the level of the signifier, this has been a very powerful model. What it cannot account for, however, is the generation of meaning (in any other than an iconographical way) or the development of a sense of familiarity, except through repetition. In short, there is no place for the reflexive subject in this model, no explanation for the generation of the sense of personal space. That is to say, in a phenomenological sense, there is no way of accounting for 'being there' except as repetition. The space of our being-there is, on the contrary, the potential space of iteration and rumination,

move and look – and that void, that penetrating, linear, inaccessible emptiness at the spatial centre of the building.

When the exhibits are in place, they will constitute the detail of these 'discursive' transients. They will be the raw data, the perceptions, the colour, the fragmentary remains, the cultural phonemes out of which one will seek to imagine the Jews in Germany/Berlin. The building is intended as a hieroglyph of the geography of Jewish Berlin, but the incisions that gesture towards the old haunts of that geography are eternally barred. There is no Rosetta Stone, no roster of celebrity, no map for decoding, no kidding; there is no way back. Yet, by virtue of the form

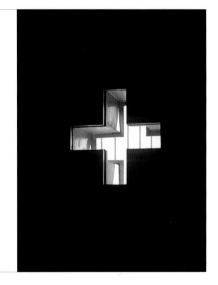

The Jewish Museum, despite its irregular form and despite the graphic style in which it has been published, is an architecturally simple, straightforward building. In its 'literal' form, it is not dissimilar to an office building.

the space of what Freud referred to as the 'phantasy-life of the individual (wherein) real internal and external sensations are interpreted and represented to himself in his mind under the influence of the pleasure-pain principle.'[2]

The Jewish Museum, despite its irregular form and despite the graphic style in which it has been published, is as stated above, an architecturally simple, straightforward building. There are no shifts in section or plan. Unlike many 'deconstructive' architectural projects, this architecture involves no decentring of the architectural signifier, no systematic exposition of the paradigmatic set of compositional possibilities. There is not even much difference in room size, not to mention any differentiation in scale, height, etc for the collections, no vistas within the volume, no moment of collective resolution. All there is, is the stark distinction between the irregular 'discursive' path of the observer, between the irregular, discursive display of the fragmentary exhibits to come, between an interrupted/ fragmented gaze – that is, the 'way' in and through which one might

of the building, the exhibits will be organised in such a way that our very movement and encounter with them will seem to echo the random character or juxtaposition, the ordinary chaos of events in everyday life. Libeskind tells us that in the basement the junctions of corridors are intended to evoke the street. But synthesis of meaning will not be satisfactory for anyone, for any imaginary coherence with which we might temporarily embellish this incompleteness will be resisted by the persistent intrusion of that void – that nothingness – emblematic of dead persons, dead, evacuated cultural niches, dead, lost artefacts, of that void, indeed, within us – a void that has the effect of reorienting us back to our desire to fabricate stories, to fill in the gap.

Libeskind refers to the theme of the building as 'between the lines'. It is a colloquialism, referring to a mode of reading in which the inferred objective of a statement is not literally articulated. What is meant is not represented or, perhaps, is inversely represented. In this instance, a narrative of the history of the 'Jewish' population of Berlin and Germany is articulated figuratively, as an absence. It is not a place for the Cartesian subject, the one who moves irregularly,

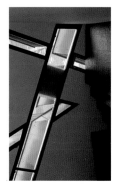

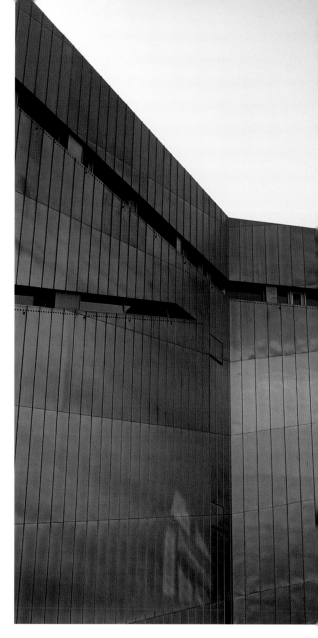

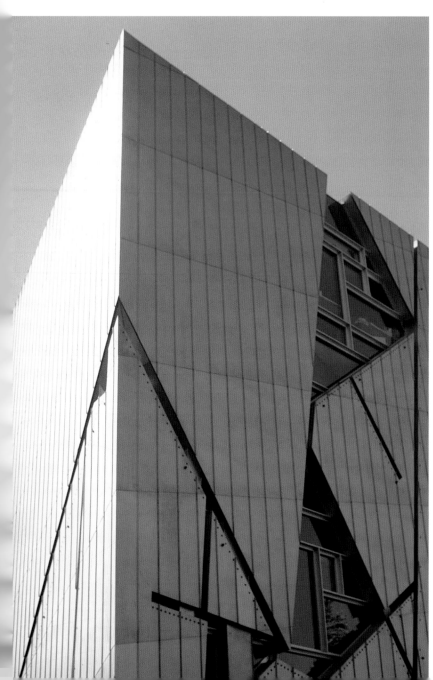

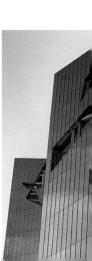

yet by the constancy of the *cogito* against the guiding, orienting rationality of an architecture, maintains narrative continuity. For in this place, the architecture is that discursive movement, that is to say, it adopts the structure of a 'subject' itself, it 'acts' as parallel witness, as interlocutor, its substance, its particulars, set against that void.

We may tear from Žižek something of what we mean by a mirroring of the subject in this interlocutionary structure:

> The Hegelian subject, ie what Hegel designates as absolute, self-relating negativity – is nothing but the very gap which separates phenomena from the Thing, the abyss beyond phenomena conceived in its negative mode, ie, the purely negative gesture of limiting phenomena without providing any positive content which would fill out the space beyond the limit.[3]

part of us at a time when the Word has been everywhere reduced to kitsch.

At the end of the tour, everyone returns to the basement, to the 'streets' and to the Holocaust Tower, which is at an extreme end of one of the corridors. The tower is entered through a door with a substantial draught seal, which sounds with an industrial or institutional 'pop' as it is opened. The architecture of the tower confirms the impersonality of the threshold, seeming to be just a bit of industrial engineering – the Jacob's ladder higher up – a duct, maybe, concrete, narrow and several storeys high, but with a bright light at its apex contrasting with the relative darkness below. It is a warm, sunny day and the guide apologises, noting that it would be a better experience if the day had been dark and cold. But the weather is no index of horror. Neither, in this most poignant of spaces, could any iconography have registered the terrifying proximity of the horror all the more explicitly.

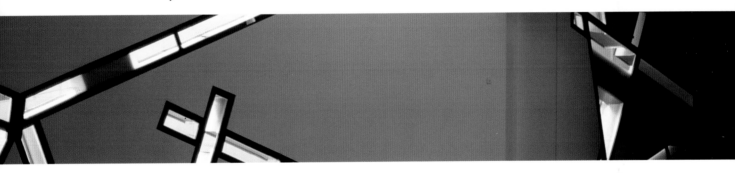

The void, in this instance the 'museum', is the very figure of the subject, the 'thing that thinks … that very "nothing", the purely formal void which is left over after the substantial content has wholly "passed over" into its predicates-determinations'.[4]

It is the void, not as representation but as actual, persistent nagging, which transforms the otherwise merely catalogued 'formal-logical network' of this architecture into a form of dialogue. The possibility of entering into this dialogue exists only in the impossibility of entering the volume of that irruptive void. We enter into the knowledge and understanding of the 'objects' to which this building is dedicated, not just in the recognition of the impossibility of our contemplation of them in their totality, but in the actual impossibility of our concrete-direct experience of them for what they putatively are. Indeed, they are a hallucination to the extent that we will look at them in the knowledge that they signify, stand for, something that was voided, a project that was never completed, a project that in terms of its desire was violently cancelled. Hence, the building can 'speak' directly to some

All is still. The guide speaks with precisely enunciated sound, pronunciation effected mostly by the lips, cheeks and tongue to accompanying, similarly abrupt and subtle, bodily punctuation. But although the body movements are timed to verbal syllables, they are not correlated to discourse, but are simply minor adjustments of balance. I can hear my heartbeat, hear the tingle of blood around my ears. The concrete appears soft and grey on this most comfortable of days. There is a short interval. The door is opened.

After leaving the Holocaust Tower, we traverse the stylised streets and go back, out to an exit point and into the ETA Hoffmann Garden, the Garden of Exile and Remembrance. It is good to be outside. The garden is made up of a series of concrete shafts (the inverse of the Holocaust Tower), which rise to an equal height in a grid pattern on plan. The most striking thing is that they all lean at the same slight angle, and are planted at the top with olive trees; light green leaves and blue sky making an inaccessible forest canopy. Visually it is even pretty – light green leaves, blue sky, peaceful modern sculpture – but within it is a labyrinth of a mildly dizzying sensation in the loss of the vertical. It is a sense of not being there. The Garden of Exile. I am relieved to be alive, somewhere. Haunted. Δ

Notes
1. Robert Young, *Mental Space*, Process Press (London), 1994, p 121.
2. Ibid, p 80.
3. Slavoj Žižek, *Tarrying with the Negative, Kant, Hegel, and the Critique of Ideology*, Duke University Press (Durham), 1993, p 21.
4. Ibid, p 80.

Reconstructing Recollection

Making Space for Memory

Memorials to the Holocaust in Israel are more than a form of remembrance dedicated to its victims, for they are historically linked with the founding of the state. More explicitly than elsewhere, the function of the museum is, as described by Yael Padan, to keep the 'Holocaust alive' as a part of the Israeli 'narrative'. Whereas the use of the word 'tragic' is frequent in these discussions, in this particular instance it could be no more distant from its classical antecedent. Whereas the function of tragedy was to arrive at a position of closure, where nothing further would be possible, that is, to structure an *action* without a future, the function of the Holocaust museum or memorial in Israel is, according to Padan, to forge a memory of the holocaust 'that cannot or should not be reused for remembering other material', that is, to create an *image* without a future.

Preserving the memory of the Holocaust is becoming an increasingly important issue as distance grows from the event itself, and survivors and witnesses age and die. What had in the past been part of everyday life in Israel, where memory was passed on by the survivors themselves, must now become an organised collective experience if it is to be remembered. The memory of the Holocaust in Israel has an additional importance: it forms a fundamental part of the Israeli national narrative. Hence, the current increase in buildings and monuments devoted to the memory of the Holocaust, commissioned by Yad Vashem – the Holocaust Martyrs and Heroes Remembrance Authority – as well as by survivors' organisations. These monuments raise some interesting questions regarding the role of architecture as repository for collective memory. What is the function of architecture in the process of institutionalising and replacing living memory? What kind of memory will be shaped into built form, and for which purpose? In what ways can buildings convey these abstract messages?

However, the choice of architecture did not assume a connection between the contents of memory and the buildings. On the contrary, the same set of spaces could be reused for remembering different materials, because the contents of memory were less fixed in the mind than the visual image of places.[1]

The contemporary Holocaust museum can be viewed as a built container for memories, an architectural attempt to create a device meant to generate recollection. However, the link between spatial experiences in the building and memory is not intended to be merely coincidental or functional. It tries to give memory a distinctive shape; one that cannot or should not be reused for remembering other materials. Two recently completed memorials and one educational building in Israel are interesting examples of different approaches to the role of architecture in giving shape to collective memory. These are Yad Layeled, the Children's Memorial Museum, by Ram Karmi and Partners; the Valley of the Communities by Dan Zur and Lippa Yahalom; and the International School for Holocaust Studies by Guggenheim\Bloch Architects and Urbanists (David Guggenheim, Alex Bloch and Daniel Mints).

The museum or memorial is intended to create a setting for the projection of memory on to a built form, providing a new linkage between memory and space.

The memory of events of communal importance is usually associated with the places in which they occurred, linking collective memory with specific spatial frameworks. However, in the case of Israel, temporal distance from the events is coupled with physical distance from the sites of occurrence, leaving memory in the realm of narrative, with no specific location. The museum or memorial is intended to create a setting for the projection of memory on to a built form, providing a new linkage between memory and space. This type of projection has been explored by Frances Yates in her book *The Art of Memory* (1966), a study of a system first developed by the ancient Greeks. The art of memory was based on the assumption that visual images are most easily remembered, and therefore the subjects of remembrance should be memorised together with familiar architectural spaces. These could later be revisited in the mind, evoking recollection.

Yad Layeled, the Children's Memorial Museum, is located at the Ghetto Fighters' Kibbutz in the north of Israel, a kibbutz founded by Holocaust survivors, ghetto fighters and partisans. The building stands in an open field at the edge of a Roman aqueduct, and is entered from the top level. Inside, a spiral exhibition ramp descends around a central cone on which the names of children are inscribed. The external wall has no openings and daylight enters the building from a skylight around the cone. Hence, the exhibition ramp seems to take the visitor into the earth, disconnected from place and time. At the end of this descent there is a metaphorical leap back to the present – the visitor exits the building, moving from its lowest point, which is dimly lit by a candle, to the contrasting brightness of the landscape outside.

The memory device used by the architect is a symbolic route in which recollection is introduced to the body through the spiral movement downwards. This is an architectural interpretation of a journey to another realm in which the world outside becomes irrelevant.

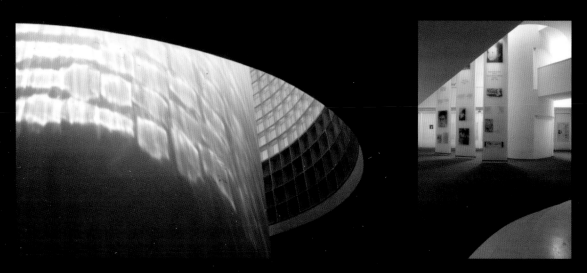
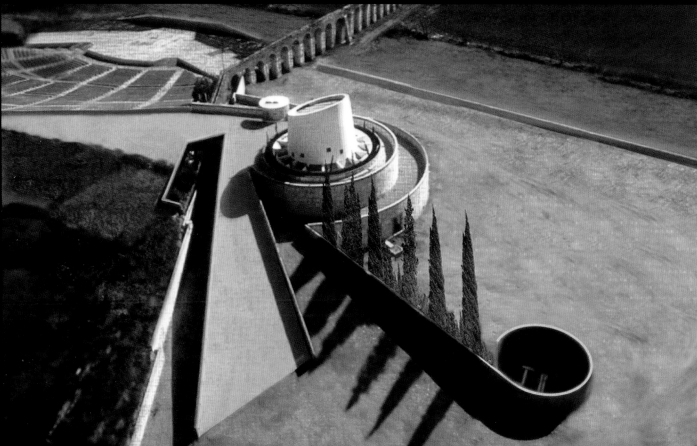
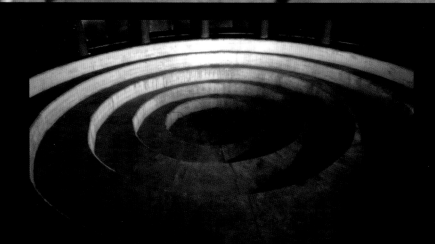

Circulation inside the building is of utmost importance, determined by a strict configuration that leads the visitor down in a single one-way route. Its linearity is further emphasised by the symbolic exit from darkness into the light of the external world. This approach brings to mind a powerful description of Auschwitz by the writer Yehiel Dinur, known as *ka-tzetnik* 135633 (concentration camp inmate No 135633). He described it as a different planet, the planet of ashes, where there were different laws of nature and a different time prevailed. But the planet of ashes still faces and affects planet earth.[2]

Perhaps because this building is associated with children, it lends a very simple architectural shape to collective memory. This shape guides the visitor into a predetermined architectural experience of movement and light that has a strong perceptual impact on the senses. Moreover, by its distinct geometry, the building conducts the visitor to a definite conclusion. The contents of this conclusion are, however, didactic and therefore beyond the realm of architecture. 'The historical memory of Yad Layeled has left a mark on the Israeli identity. The greatest challenge of the post-Holocaust generation is to preserve and rebuild our Jewish identity', wrote architect Ram Karmi about his museum.[3] This approach views the building narrowly as a tool for reinforcing the Israeli narrative: since we the Jews were victims of anti-Semitism and its unparalleled crimes, our collective memory of this trauma may now be shaped to strengthen our national identity. On the other hand, the curator Miri Kedem expresses a more universal view of the dangers of racism. She writes of the human capacity to cause suffering, regardless of race and nation, when she describes the period of the Holocaust as one 'in which one part of mankind was losing its humanity, while the other was paying the unbearable price, yet remaining human'.[4]

Yad Vashem was established in 1953 by a special act of the Israeli parliament. Its 45 acre site in Jerusalem, Har Hazikaron (the Mount of Remembrance), is one of the fundamental locations of Israeli collective identity, visited by all official guests of the state of Israel. It includes a historical museum, an art museum, different outdoor monuments, the Valley of the Communities and research and educational institutes including the International School for Holocaust Studies. The annual Holocaust Martyrs and Heroes Remembrance Day is opened by an official ceremony there, followed by a special educational programme in all the country's schools. Most visitors to Yad Vashem are therefore aware beforehand of the contents and meaning of the site.

The Valley of the Communities is a labyrinthine shape dug into the ground and open to the sky, with walls of rock, almost 9 metres high, carrying the names of every Jewish community destroyed in the Holocaust. Its plan roughly resembles a map of Central and Eastern Europe, with the names carved more or less according to their geographical location. The size of each community is indicated by different fonts. The visitor wanders in and out of spaces in a strange landscape, surrounded by the massive walls that block all views except the sky, and by thousands of names.

The configuration of this monument refers directly to geography, giving an almost literal expression to the idea of creating a location for memory. The walls of rock enclose the visitor on the floor of a symbolic excavation, creating an artificial site of archaeology. The inscriptions, part epitaph, part ancient engraving, create an almost primeval memory. In this sense, this site too is disconnected from the outside world, but here the seemingly abstract setting actually represents real places that have been scaled down and condensed. Hence, the visitor is lost in a sunken labyrinth, but at the same time some sense of orientation is provided by the opportunity to locate a specific community name in relation to others. The combination of an abstracted pit with an actual landscape is therefore effective on two levels. One is the immediate sense of dislocation and insecurity, experienced whether or not the visitor is familiar with the map of Europe. The other is based on knowledge and recognition of the logic of movement inside the maze.

The approach to commemoration in this structure does not appeal to a sense of identification with the story of an individual or a community. Rather, it deals with the aspect of numbers. One of the difficulties in representing the memory of the Holocaust is its scope, since the immense numbers of victims and sites make them impossible to grasp. In the Valley of the Communities the architects have used scale as a memory device, giving a notion of the relative location and size of the Jewish communities as an indication to the number of victims. At the same time, the size of this scaled-down space itself creates a new imagined landscape, on which memory is literally imprinted.

The International School for Holocaust Studies differs from the two other projects in that it is neither a museum nor a memorial. It contains 17 classrooms and different educational facilities including an auditorium and multimedia and resource centres. In addition, there are offices and research rooms. The building is three storeys high, traversed by one long, open space. Light enters through a skylight over this space, and through huge windows facing the landscape of Jerusalem on

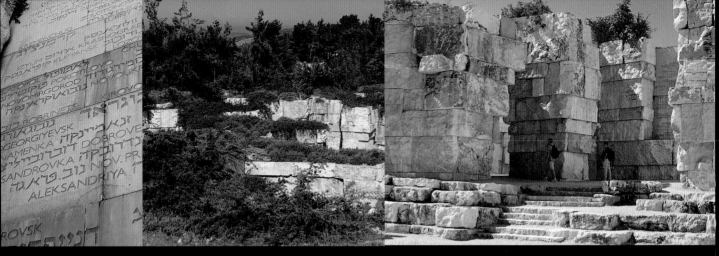

Above
**Valley of the Communities by
Dan Zur and Lippa Yahalom**

Above left
The names of thousands of
Jewish communities destroyed
in the Holocaust are carved
in the rock walls.

Above middle
Sunk into the ground like an
ancient excavation site, the
Valley of the Communities is
barely visible from a distance.

Above right
Within the maze of rocks
and names.

Right
**The International School
for Holocaust Studies**
by Guggenheim\Bloch
Architects and Urbanists,
David Guggenheim,
Alex Bloch, Daniel Mints

Top left
Exterior view of
pedagogic library.

Top right
View of central void.

Bottom left
View of main stair.

Bottom right
View of breaking point
of the main axis.

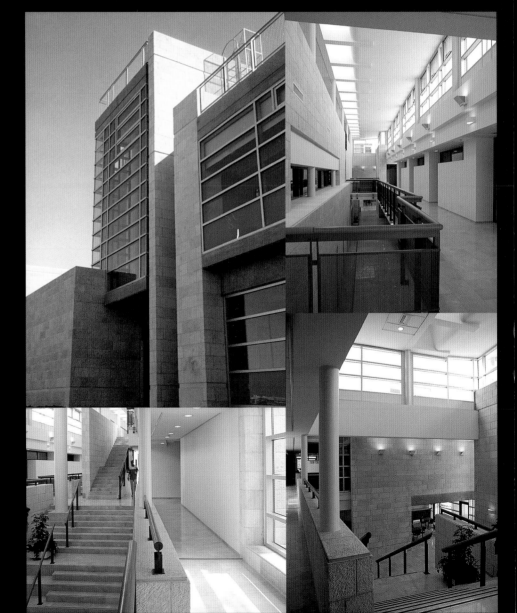

Architecture in this building explicitly addresses its specific site. The visitor is not detached from the outside world but is constantly aware of its presence, even inside the classrooms. Symbolic elements are subtle and abstracted.

one side of the building and small courtyards on the other. Most of the circulation in the different levels of the building occurs in the central space. Staff quarters are arranged on one side, classrooms on the other, providing a clear sense of orientation.

Architecture in this building explicitly addresses its specific site. The visitor is not detached from the outside world but is constantly aware of its presence, even inside the classrooms. Symbolic elements are subtle and abstracted. The central space uniting all functions is a void, figuratively a container of time, represented by the changing conditions of natural light. The central stair marks a breaking point in the directionality of the axis, before revealing the view through the huge glass wall of the cafeteria. The remaining axis ends symbolically with a window facing a stone wall.

The notion reflected in this building is that education is a long and lasting process, whose contents have no explicit configuration for they lie in the realm of narrative. Hence its architecture does not attempt to shape collective memory by using distinctive geometry or isolation from reality to give the visitor an immediate experience of recollection. Rather,

the building is a container for knowledge, providing admirable surroundings for study and contemplation, and in this sense it could have been any kind of educational institute. Its location at Yad Vashem provides sufficient background for its purpose, freeing the building of excessive symbolism, and emphasising the importance of the conceptual contents of collective memory.

The three sites reviewed here present very different perceptions of architecture as a holder and generator of collective memory. As the temporal gap widens, the importance of architecture in giving narrative a fixed shape increases. An intelligible spatial experience is associated with the contents of memory in an organised process of recollection, somewhat in the mode of the art of memory. However, all three projects reveal the intricacy of trying to give physical expression to the memory of the Holocaust, as well as the limitations of architecture as narrative. It is now our responsibility to contemplate the contents of memory and to determine which of its aspects have been presented to us. The question remains to what extent is the visitor being directed towards collective memory, whether national or universal, and what is the meaning of its conclusions in Israel? Do we remember the horrors of the Holocaust as victims only, or are we still aware of the world outside these monuments? ⊅

Notes
1. Frances A Yates, *The Art of Memory*, Penguin Books (London), 1966.
2. *The General Attorney Versus Adolph Eichman: Testimonies*, Israeli Centre for Information, 1963, p 1122 (published in Hebrew).
3. See Yad Layeled website: www.ghf.org.il.
4. Ibid.

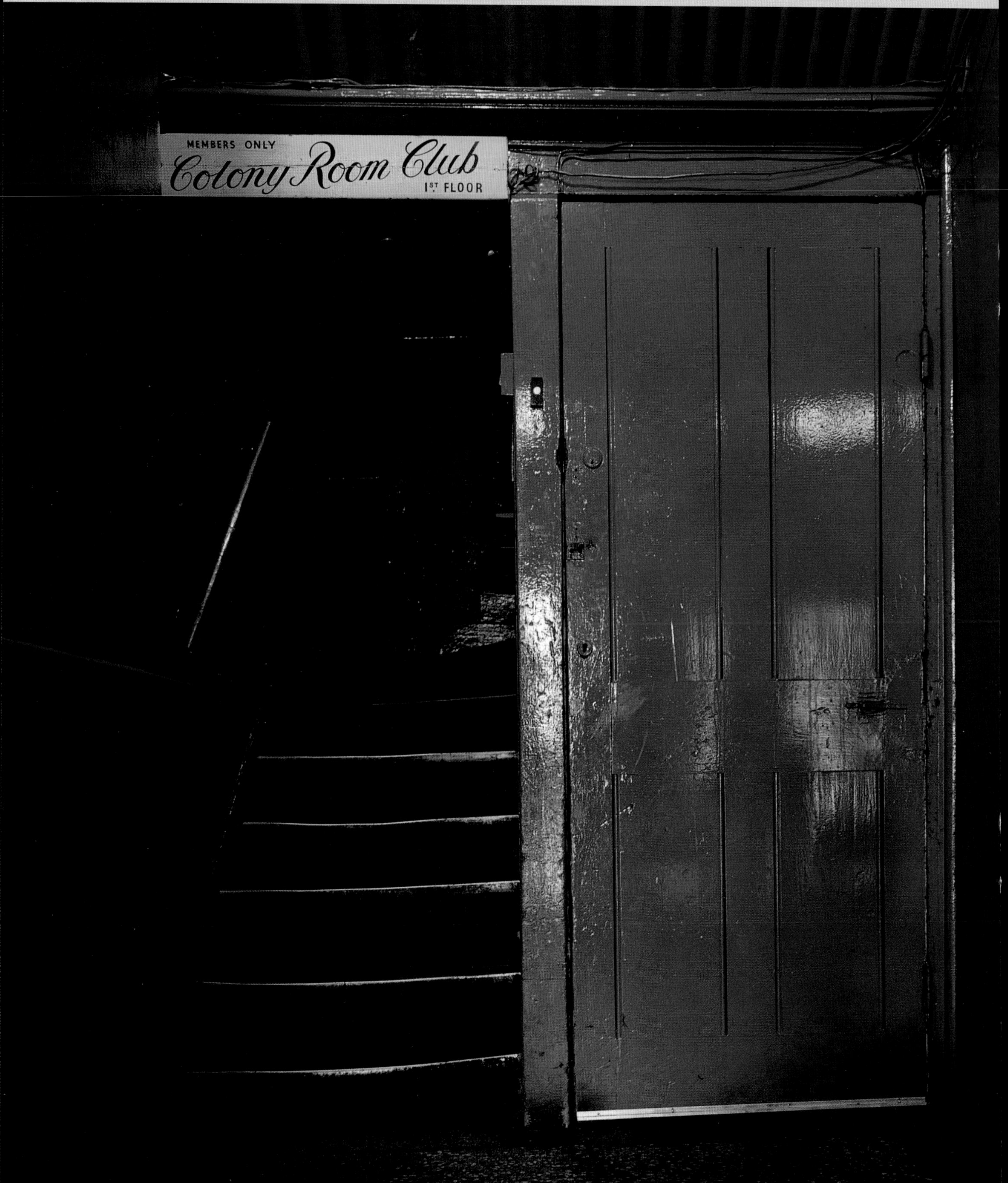
MEMBERS ONLY
Colony Room Club
1ST FLOOR

Sacraria, Tragedy and the

Interior Narrative

Tragic themes involving the confrontation of heroic actions with a malevolent fate have no purchase on the frustrations of everyday life and melancholic loss. There is little in the everyday use of terms to distinguish tragedy from mere pathos, and indeed it is in this way that we normally hear use of the term. In his examination of the exceptional nature of sacred spaces within the context of modernity, Edward Winters confronts the sadness of contemporary subjective aspiration. Developing his argument against the possibility of direct expression or narrative in architecture, it is nonetheless uncertain, by these criteria that the creation even of void space for habitation by 'the sacred Thing' may be carried out with any greater certainty.

The job of the theorist teaching in a school of architecture is to reflect upon the character of architecture taken at its broadest. The theorist tries best to smooth things out when thought gets crumpled and creased in the puzzles, muddles and confusions that arise naturally from consideration of what architecture is or what it ought to be. Is there a language of architecture? Is architecture a fine art? Is architecture a representational art? Or is it expressive? And so on. In answering this kind of question, the theorist draws upon resources developed in epistemology, philosophy of mind, philosophy of language and, of course, aesthetics. Answers to these very general questions then provide insights upon which we can call in our answers to other more specific questions, such as: in what way can architecture be thought tragic?

Architecture is not a representational art.[1] Like music, it is abstract. Tragedy, by contrast, is a mode of narrative found only in the representational arts. How then are we to understand the claim that architecture might be tragic? Here we might profit by shifting our focus from the stuff of architecture (bricks and mortar) and concentrating instead on the kind of experience to which architecture typically gives rise.

We should resist the view, prevalent in much modernist thought, that it is to form that we attend when considering works of architecture. Architecture, although an abstract art, is not merely the composition of elements considered as lines, volumes, shapes, colours, textures and spaces. Such compositions are compatible only with the free judgements of beauty, where the object of appreciation is allowed to float free from any determining concept. Kant, whose work inspired and supported formalist aesthetics, expressly denies this formal approach to the appreciation of architecture, pointing up the difference between free and dependent beauty thus:

> When we judge free beauty (according to mere form) then our judgement of taste is pure. Here we presuppose no concept of any purpose ... and hence no concept (as to) what the object is (meant) to represent; our imagination is playing, as it were, while it contemplates the shape, and such a concept would only restrict its freedom.[2]

> By contrast, the beauty of a horse or of a building (such as a church, palace, armoury or summer-house) does presuppose the concept of the purpose that determines what the thing is (meant) to be, and hence a concept of its perfection.[3]

Whilst the notion of free beauty remains – for this reader at least – irredeemably obscure, it is clear that for Kant the beauty of architecture is a dependent beauty. It depends upon our conception of the building under view as a work of architecture. And further, we might think, the conception of the particular circumstances of the work will enter into our consideration of it – that it is a village church, or that it faces on to a public square. The projected use of a building and its relationships to other buildings (and their uses) enter into our judgements of works of architecture. Unlike buildings, however, our lives do have a narrative dimension. And so it is in the lived relationship between built form and the lives of those who inhabit that form that we might hope to project narrative content. It is content that, whilst belonging to a living community, connects with the symbolic function of architecture. It is such content that might invest architecture with the quality of tragedy. In particular, where we expect to find prescribed ritual and its attendant symbolism in architecture, we might thereby expect to find something approaching narrative form.

An obvious place to start is in church. The liturgy of the Mass, with all its paraphernalia, its processions and its repetitions, is fabricated in sacred form. The queue to take the Eucharist, the queue to make reconciliation in the confessional, the side chapels with their patron saints, and the stations of the cross, all require processional form. The light from the rose window or from the lanterned dome exists outside the temporal narrative of the procession and bathes worshippers in eternal light. And so one function of the architecture provides a counterpoint to another; and thereby provides the occasion upon which to think about the nature of human life and its episodes *sub specie aeternitatis*.

Moreover, a duty of the Church is to remind us of our condition and to provide us with hope for atonement, redemption and salvation. The prayer to Our Lady implores her to 'Pray for us sinners, Now and at the hour of our death'. Hence, we are to connect our selves now to our selves projected forward to the scenes of our deathbeds. Alone amongst creation we are conscious of our mortality. This is our tragedy. Christ's was to have suffered crucifixion unto death for our sins and to have felt forsaken by God at that hour. The hope of triumph over tragedy is the resurrection. However, it is a modern tragedy that the narrative of Christ's passion has come to be regarded as a metaphor as opposed to a literal, if mysterious, truth. Science and Enlightenment thought have largely removed the one consolation that the Church provided. Modernist art and architecture offer evidence of our spiritual and aesthetic bereavement.

In our homes, we make interiors to accommodate the individuals we have become. As a child, I grew up with troughs for holy water by the side of each door. And every shelf, ledge and mantelpiece supported pictures of religious scenes, or small statuettes that had been collected from churches on family visits at home or abroad. In Indonesia there are little roadside shrines that make small offerings to the gods – a tinfoil cup of flowers and rice for instance. In Catholic countries throughout the world we see flowers and photographs, small symbolic images put together in remembrance of some lost loved one. These are *sacraria* – sacred spaces designed to house the spirit of the lost or the dead. In the reliquary tradition, humble objects are invested with meaning by their association with the soul for whom the shrine has been created. A room, a space, a box, a tinfoil cup of rice can become a sacrarium. The scenes of grief and the heap of flowers outside Kensington Palace following the death of Princess Diana are testimony to the fact that ordinary people still seek this symbolism.

Joseph Cornell created tragic interiors whose magic spaces serve to connect us with a sense of the sacred. There is a feeling of both love and loss in his works and, when seen as rooms, they can provide much by way of inspiration for a new conception of architectural significance. My own work as an artist, developed in the context of an architecture school, is influenced by Cornell and by the search to provide sacred spaces with something akin to poetic narrative.

Elsewhere, we find interiors that reflect upon our tragic condition and that connect with the kind of sensitivity which I have been adverting to. The time we waste in bars bears witness to a sort of longing that might once have been ministered to by the Church. Geoffrey Firmin, an alcoholic British consul in Malcolm Lowry's *Under the Volcano*, is drinking and writing a letter to his estranged wife, Yvonne:

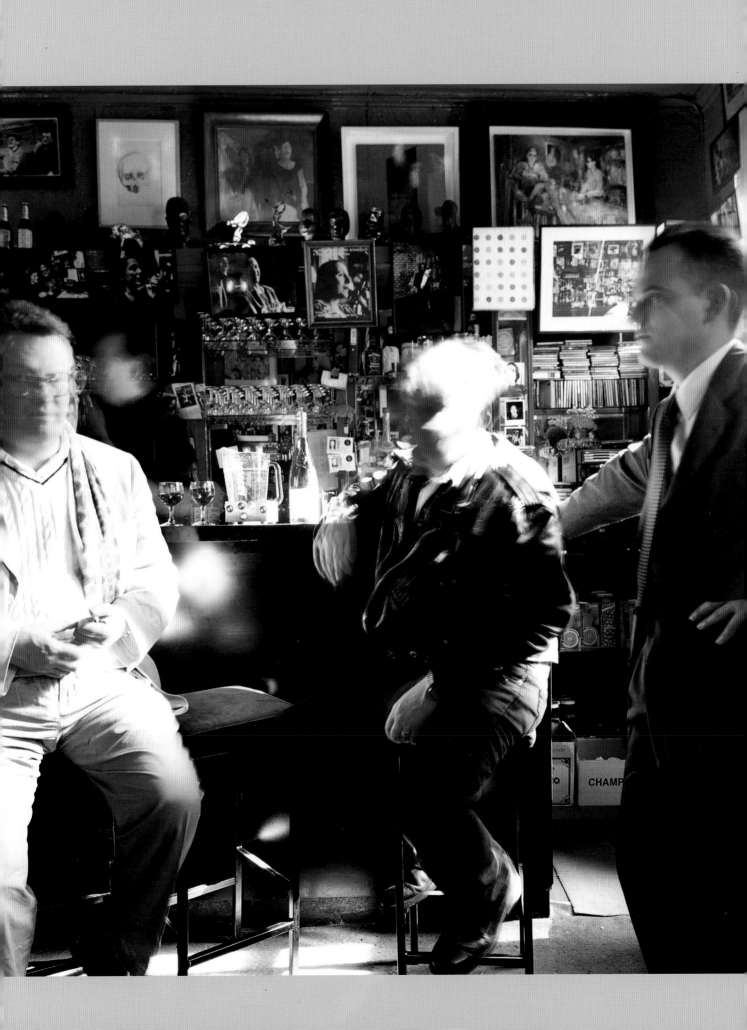

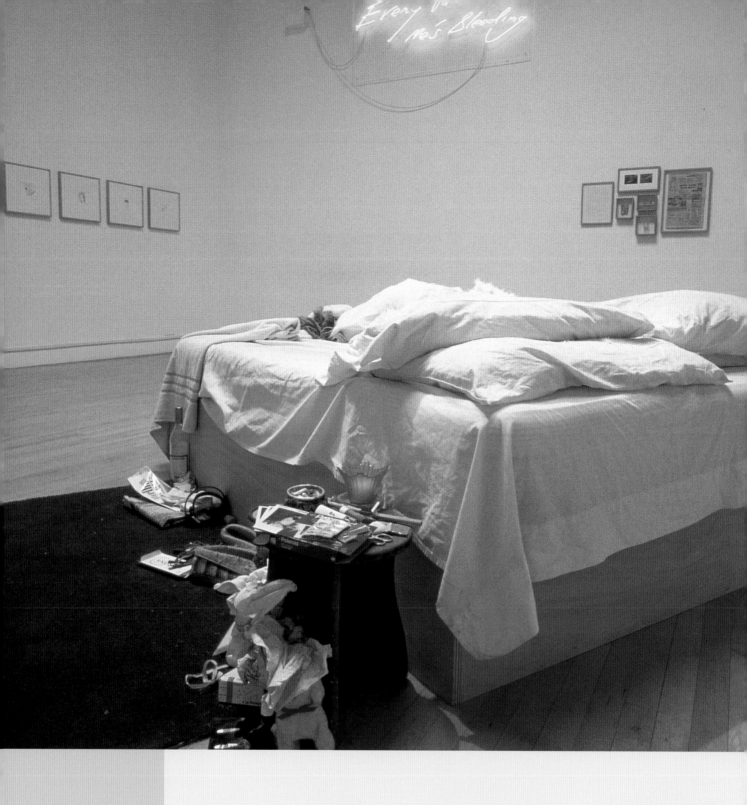

Above
Tracey Emin, *My Bed*,
installation, Tate Gallery,
London, 1998 (mattress,
linens, pillows, rope and
various memorabilia,
79 x 211 x 234 cm).

Bottom left
Edward Winters, Vanessa,
mixed media, 1986.

Bottom middle
Edward Winters, Lie there with
Rosie, mixed media, 1998,
collection Colony Room Club.

Bottom right
Edward Winters, Dark Angel,
mixed media, 2000.

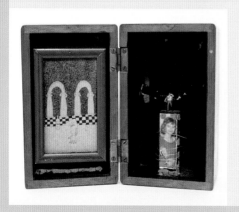 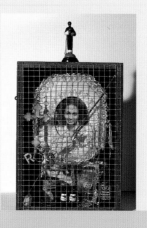 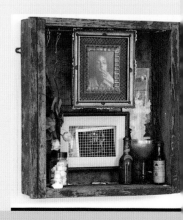

Hers is a postfeminist expression of tragedy in the failure of modern love. Hers is an art of narrative that cries out for salvation in an otherwise dismal world.

Love is the only thing that gives meaning to our poor ways on earth: not precisely a discovery, I am afraid. You will think I am mad, but this is how I drink too, as if I were taking an eternal sacrament.[4]

And in the next chapter:

(Y)ou misunderstand me if you think it is altogether darkness I see, and if you insist on thinking so, how can I tell you why I do it? But if you look at that sunlight there, ah, then perhaps you'll get the answer, see, look at the way it falls through the window: what beauty can compare to that of a cantina in the early morning? ... (T)hink of all the other terrible (cantinas) where people go mad that will soon be taking down their shutters, for not even the gates of heaven, opening wide to receive me, could fill me with such celestial complicated and hopeless joy as the iron screen that rolls up with a crash, as the unpadlocked jostling jealousies which admits those whose souls tremble with the drinks they carry unsteadily to their lips. All mystery, all hope, all disappointment, yes, all disaster, is here beyond those swinging doors ... How, unless you drink as I do, can you hope to understand the beauty of an old woman from Tarasco who plays dominoes at seven o'clock in the morning?[5]

The Colony Room Club in Soho has for 50 years been a bar in which Bohemians can waste away the hours, drinking recklessly and watching the sun flood in from south-facing first-floor windows. Once, it was home to Francis Bacon, to others of the London School, and to any number of lesser known artists, all of whom would have been familiar with Lowry's novel and the tragedy it expressed. Today, it has embraced a younger set of artists including Damien Hirst, Mark Quinn and Tracey Emin. The club itself retains the air of a sacred space, the generations mixing like those at Mass who turn to give each other a sign of friendship.

Tracey Emin's *Bed* (1999) extends the thread of work of which I have been writing. Perhaps the Expressionism to which she is given – with its overtly sexual content – could only be promulgated by a woman. Hers is a postfeminist expression of tragedy in the failure of modern love. Hers is an art of narrative that cries out for salvation in an otherwise dismal world. Like others before, she uses the reliquary tradition to invoke meaning, significance and a sense of awe. Because she is a woman, she is able to force us to confront the hopelessness of erotic love in our postmodern lives. (If a man were to do this, it would look bombastic or sentimental; or both.) But hers is the kind of art that makes for interior spaces and the sacred nature of spaces to which I have been alluding. That there is the possibility to explore human tragedy within the context of the architectural interior is something that seems to me to provide hope. It is only by facing full square the tragic nature of our lives that we can come to grasp the nature of hope. And then we shall require an architecture that embodies this.

Of course, the architecture of the city – an urban design – might well be thought to provide the context for another kind of interior narrative. The interior of the city, developed from the view I have been putting forward here, might generate a new kind of architecture made to accommodate the narrative of lives and sensitivities of a people in search of the spiritual. ◬

Notes
1. I have argued for this against Nelson Goodman's semantic theory, and against both the souvenir theory and the classicist mimetic theory in 'Architecture Meaning and Significance', *The Journal of Architecture*, vol 1, no 1, Spring 1996.
2. Immanuael Kant, *The Critique of Judgement*, trans Werner S Pluhar, Hackett (Indianapolis), 1987, 1 #16, p 77.
3. Ibid.
4. Malcolm Lowry, *Under The Volcano*, Jonathan Cape (London), 1967, p 40.
5. Ibid, p 50.

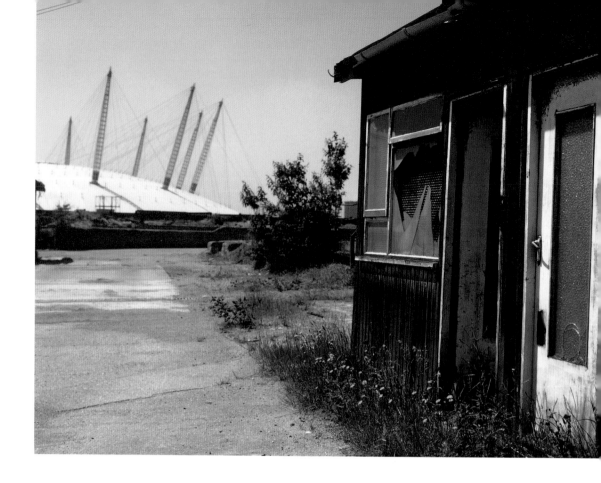

Sitting in the White Horse, Thinking about a White Elephant

The foreclosure of the tragic, of the mythic and symbolic, the casting of spirit into the maelstrom of history may be listed amongst the most definitive of figures in modernity. Yet 'tragedy' at large is something of a weapon used to capture the miserable frustrations of everyday life and worse. Is it reasonable to correlate the death of tragedy with the decline of civic rectitude? Can we pick up any facts, lying about as facts do, that might assist us in coming to a reasonable judgement on such a question? Are there any major symbolic projects around by which we might test these things? Is London's Millennium Dome tragic? Of course not. Does it aspire to great themes? Of course not. Is it the epitome of the mechanical construction of 'space'? Does it span the gap, the literal void between the technological provision of amenity and individual dreams and obsessions? Paul Davies tells us something of the life from which it sprang.

Everybody asks me when, exactly, I knew the Dome was going to be a disaster. The truth is, I still don't know if it is. A bit of me thought it would be a disaster from the word go, from that first meeting around a big conference table gulping white wine opposite a highly argumentative eco-warrior. But by the first half-term holiday of 2000, with parents desperate to find something to do with the kids, and a man from Disney at the helm, the Dome was crowded out. Not that popularity is necessarily the best criterion for judging success until you consider all the others.

Success was the last thing on my mind when, at lunchtime on a grey February day in 2000, I walked through the side entrance of the White Horse on Shoreditch High Street. The place gives little away from the outside, except for the multicoloured chalk lettering advertising 'Exotic Dancers'. Some architect, some latter-day Borromini, should have made something of it, that transformation from mundane street to wanton interior. If the dancers were making the effort, exchanging their everyday attire of duffel coats and back packs for a pair of £120, 6 inch high heels in glitter Perspex, and a sexy outfit of blue tasselled stretch-something from their personal tailor up the street, that modest little doorway wasn't exactly doing much to help them.

Inside, 'Monster Trucks' flickered on the screen behind the corner stage. Above it, supporting seven storeys of masonry, big downstand beams fanned out from the corner of the bar, which, this early, saw just a few regulars reading their papers, and the girls waltzing around, precariously balanced on stilettos, all smiles, waiting for the rush of suits. I was feeling sentimental, for this big cherry-wood room had always been a good place to think, and was where, between live dancers and taped disasters, bloopers and funnies, a large percentage of my work on the Dome was done.

I had ordered twice before Gaby, naked by now, did the splits and everybody winced. The prospect of a lost afternoon of sitting in the White Horse, thinking about a white elephant was on the cards.

Back in our heyday, 1998, when I first began collaborating with Tim Pyne, principal designer of WORK, this was our design studio where watching striptease, own goals, scooting poodles, catastrophic ski runs, Benny Hill skits, female wrestlers in feathers, cowgirl boxers, or boxing nurses was, compared to everything else, good honest entertainment; a place where you could learn stuff. We debated ideas amidst cheap

thrills, and delivered them in more socially advantageous venues like the Great Eastern dining rooms. It was a hell of a lot of fun.

Lesson one in this new world of the Dome: all work was social, and most of it done standing up. And my job, in comparison to all the others who really did the work on the project, was merely to chaperone ideas, or rather the irascible vessel that generated them, between venues. Riding pillion between the anonymous office block in Victoria that was the New Millennium Experience Company headquarters and Tim's white-box apartment with the single Mathew Hilton sofa that was my home for much of the time. Waking, peering through whisky hangovers, wondering where we'd been: to the office (occasionally), the Bricklayers Arms, the Reliance; from the cocoon of the Coach and Horses and back to Blacks; on Devon beaches, and in the car parks of Las Vegas casinos watching the sun rise; from switchback drives down Sunset Boulevard to the ocean; to drunken hospitality tents at Sandown Park. As I said: a hell of a lot of fun.

I had first met Tim on election night, outside a scraggy art show in Notting Hill. He looked like Austin Powers, but thought he looked like Chris Evans. He immediately struck me as the kind of person who could solve any design problem with a visit to Hamleys (which he did, on several occasions) and that he was going to do very, very well. That night, everybody was getting off on either the New Labour government or with each other over lukewarm bottles of Becks. The world, they said, would change.

Cut to three months later: after a very late night drinking in the Troy Club in Soho, Tim would split from his long-term girlfriend and leave his beloved houseboat with nothing but a Waitrose carrier bag. I had led him astray; I was the devil, the compadre with the fatal disease (as his next girlfriend referred to it). I got to hang around with him a lot, Sancho Panza to his Don Quixote, on his adventures designing the Government conception of 'One Amazing Day'. Tim was already pitching for Living Island, but he would also end up with three more zones: 'Work', 'Learn' and 'Shared Ground'. He started by aceing his application, placing it in an inflatable plastic container, just so it would have to rest on the top of the pile.

As I gazed at my pint, on that February day, I remembered Dome PR telling me that it would take 3.8 million more pints to fill the Dome, or that if it were inverted under Niagara Falls it would take 10 minutes to fill with water. I could remember the thrill: what would the Dome say? How would it say it? And could we have a zone please? Now, after the Dome had opened, how ill-founded that optimism seemed. The scale of the operation was valued over any content, and a *Which* report had just decreed that the 'Work' zone was full of 'irritating slogans' and that the 'Learn' zone was 'tacky'.

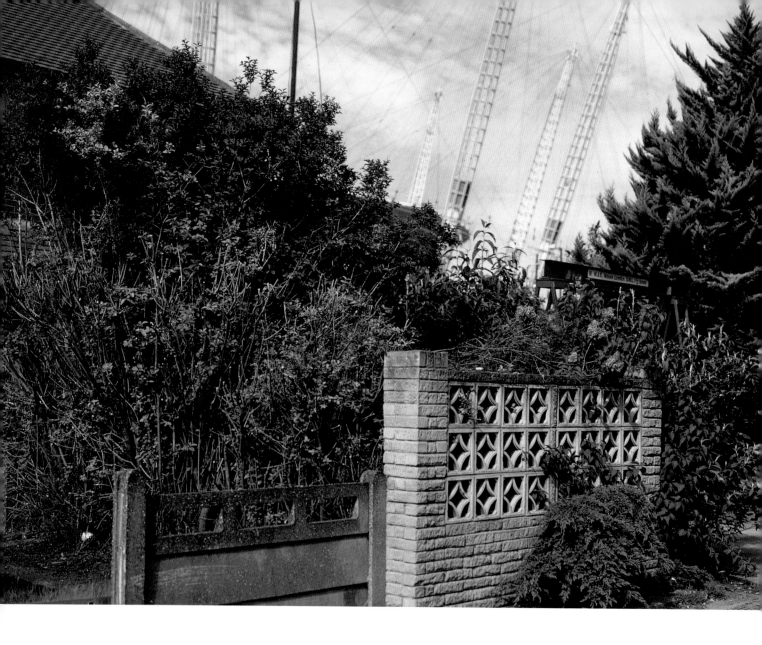

Illustrations
The Dome in context,
photographed by Jane Hamlin.

I now think Tim and I understood something, intuitively, that none of the other designers did: that if the Dome were not a museum, nor a theme park, nor a trade show, it would be a tabloid newspaper – a really good one that would be fun to read, irreverent and throwaway at the same time. Tim wanted to tell short, smart, stories. Abstractions, grandiose architectonics, funky forms were not what it was about. It was not a question of insulting the intelligence of the audience, but of empathising with them, telling personal stories, tabloid stories and building on them.

No matter that Tim lived in a white box with his *Wallpaper** magazines; he was a newshound at heart. No matter that we didn't understand, even after three months of sitting bemused with writers and researchers and sociologists and God knows who else, just what exactly was the difference between 'hard' and 'soft' skills; nor could we, for that matter, seriously contemplate a 'new' world of learning. But we could tell a story about somebody communicating well, or someone going back to college.

I remember one Sunday I got a call to the office where Tim was alone, pacing the room and staring at a weekend's drawing. His story boards for 'Learn' lined the walls, showing the unfolding memories of an old schoolmaster and the sheer numbers of individuals he had helped during his career. They were fabulous. 'This is the one! Doesn't it just make you want to cry?' Tim sparkled through tired eyes. It did, but they didn't buy it. Now that was tragic.

That office was unusual, and heaven for me, because I never knew what to do in it. Traditional design companies must have quaked when they saw it. Their overblown rosters of creatives and associated hangers-on in plush designer suites might be superbly equipped to show off cars with smoke, lasers, infinity mirrors and revolving stages, but they'd need some time in the White Horse before they could adjust to the Dome. Tim's office was a big table in a room with a few computers and a lot of mobile-phone chargers hanging from the windowsills. Later, when he needed to expand, he rented a second large room and installed a second big table and a few computers and phone chargers hanging from the sills. Tim hated those computers – this was no virtual technofantasy – but the office would slowly fill with them anyway, along with the transient collection of operatives and people who helped you through the day. There was Donut, the mild-mannered diploma grad who slumbered in tune with our hangovers; and whatsername who got the push, reluctantly (because she was really entertaining), when we discovered she'd been playing fast and loose with the company credit card down Oxford Street. I would just lie on the floor, racking my brains, or sketch out ideas in my series of little yellow notebooks, which proved highly convenient in the bar.

While I was reminiscing in the White Horse on that February day, a new team of designers had been employed to replace us on the Dome and contractors were crawling all over it, changing this and that. Presumably, they would continue to do so until it was decided to represcribe the Dome's function altogether. The sole moment of closure for the original designers was the hand over, witnessed only by insiders. Now, in any conversation about what had been done, we were all revisionists, claiming we had nothing to do with that bit or this bit as our efforts vanished before our eyes.

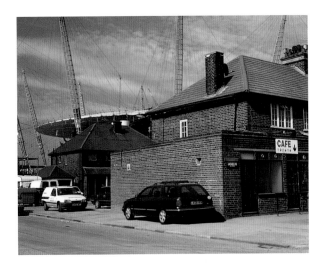

Any sense of permanence, of conceptual as well as physical solidity, is absent from the project. Aside from the ephemerality of the physical structure, the Dome was always going to be dematerialised by spin, by tabloid tactics, rather than tabloid content. Dammit, it was always going to be a white elephant, and it's just as well we had a fantastic time doing it. And the White Horse, where Shakespeare reputedly drank and just may have encountered the occasional 16th century exotic dancer, was an appropriate headquarters, beyond the prissiness of the modern designer's world.

And I had cried when I saw the 'Work' and 'Learn' shed finished, just before hand over, with all the simplicity of that little sketch in a yellow paper notebook, so smartly put together full-size by the architects Tim had contracted in to do the job. I cried because, like so many, I still betray that hopeless romanticism for the idea conceived in a bar, preferably the lowest, most ordinary bar in the whole world, accompanied by striptease. An idea that is so perfect it hardly needs to leave that room: architecture as effortlessly pleasurable and mythological as a zipless fuck.[1] ◮

Notes
1. Term coined by Erica Jong in her novel *Fear of Flying*, 1973.

Biographies
of contributors

Dr Joan R Branham is Associate Professor of Art and Architectural History at Providence College. Her publications have focused on questions of sacred space, gender, and sacrifice in Judaism and Christianity.

Helen Castle is Managing Editor of *Architectural Design.*

Paul Davies is Senior Lecturer in Architecture at South Bank University. He studied architecture at Bristol, where he specialised on the issue of sustainable construction methods. He is an unashamed populist, and an expert on Las Vegas. He was design consultant to WORK on four zones at London's Millennium Dome.

David Hamilton Eddy has written about architecture for thirty years, drawing on his interests in literature and psychology to develop his own brand of architectural criticism. Over the last ten years he has focused on Futurism, Erich Mendelsohn and American Streamlining, all in connection with his interest in curved architecture. Otherwise, he hangs out with his fictional alter ego, the Atlanta private eye, Eddie Jackson.

Dr Tim Martin is Head of Design Management at the Leicester School of Architecture, de Montford University. He has written for *The Architects' Journal*, The *British Art Journal*, and is author of *The Essential Surrealists.* He is also presenter of 'Landmarks in Western Art' for the Discovery Channel.

Robert Maxwell is an architect and former Dean of the School of Architecture at Princeton University.

John Outram is a practising architect, whose buildings make extensive use of the iconographical tradition. www.johnoutram.com/forest.html

Yael Padan is a practising Israeli architect, who studied at the Bartlett School of Architecture, University College London, obtaining an MA in History of Modern Architecture. She now writes on architectural history and theory.

Richard Patterson is an architect and Course Leader for the Diploma in Architecture at the Leicester School of Architecture. He has studied at the University of California, Cambridge University, The Architectural Association and Princeton University. His published work has been concerned with the iconography of Renaissance gardens, the language of Vitruvius and the application of psychoanalytical theory in architectural criticism.

Astrid Schmeing is a practising architect. She studied at the Fachhochschule Mnster, at the Architectural Association in London, and, as a Fulbright Scholar, at Ohio State University. She writes on German architecture and teaches at the Architectural Association and at the Technical University Karlsruhe.

Edward Winters is Senior Lecturer in the Department of Architecture at the University of Westminster. He studied painting at the Slade School before going on to read philosophy at the University of London. He has since published widely on the visual arts and has given academic papers at universities in America and Europe. He is a founder member of The Centre for Visual Culture (University of Westminster/University College London) and a practising painter.

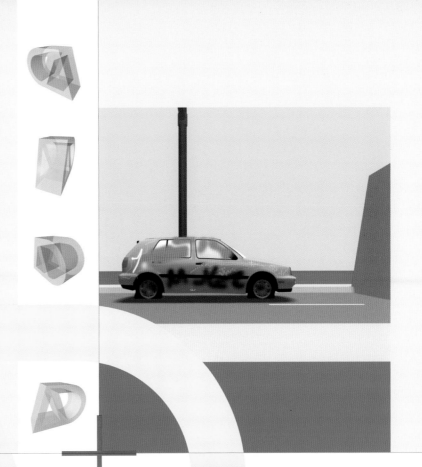

Edited by Helen Castle

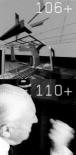

A Quiet Revolution: Women in French Practice

At a time when there should be equal opportunities in education and the profession, worldwide women are still a minority among qualified architects. Robert Such reports from France – a country which has been slow to accept women in the profession. He looks at the innovative work of Françoise-Hélène Jourda, Odile Decq and Manuelle Gautrand and explores how three highly talented French women are making it on their own.

Unlike Britain – which boasted the first female architects – the French were slower in allowing women into the club. Also noticeable by its absence has been a strong feminist movement and general lack of gender studies in the curriculum. To find the first women to receive an architecture diploma in France requires a trip back down the time line to 1901 when the American, Julia Morgan graduated from the École des Beaux Arts, three years after Ethel Mary Charles joined the RIBA. Real change in France, however, did not begin until the May 1968 student insurgency against, among other things, the archaic French university system. One result was that the teaching of architecture split off from painting and sculpture at the ancient École des Beaux Arts. From then on, the numbers of young women attending the newly created institutions steadily started to rise. However, it is worth remembering, that other areas of education still remained obstinately closed to women even after the raging street battles and sit ins. Not until 1973 did the doors of the highly regarded university, the École Polytechnique, finally swing open.

Certain activists, like that of ARVHA (Association pour la Recherche sur la Ville et l'Habitat, www.arvha.asso.fr), concerned with requalification and the NOW (New Opportunities for Women) programme, continually push for change. In 1998 NOW held the first European congress, entitled 'Women and Architecture', to tackle the issues.

Despite the fact that many women have stand alone, working couples have become widespread. Why?

'I think it's easier to work together [and] good to be able to share completely,' says Manuelle Gautrand, who brings strong designs, in the form of silk-screen printing, adhesives and graphic motifs, to her constructions. Traditional materials, resins, polycarbonates, together with transparent and translucent lighting effects, are combined with a sensitivity for context. Yet despite this desire for close co-operation, financial difficulties have meant that her husband, Marc Blaising, can only commit himself on a part-time basis. Something that she is certain will be only temporary.

Sharing and working with someone is 'enriching', agrees Odile Decq, whose partner Benoît Cornette suffered a fatal car accident in 1998. 'With Benoît, [one] had to convince the other that [something] was a good idea.' Works by Decq and Cornette include the baroque-influenced Banque Populaire de l'Ouest (1996), focusing on the passage from one area to another, a seamless slipping from place to place, and netted them ten international awards. Hypertension, an installation from 1993, further investigated perceptions of space. Through the use of reflective surfaces that inverted the observer's image, it too aimed at 'pleasurable ambiguity'.

François-Hélène Jourda
Jourda has been in independent practice for the last
five years, following her divorce from Gilles Perraudin.
Jourda-Perraudin designed the Ecole d'Architecture,
Lyon (1987). Jourda has completed the Academy of
Further Education, Herne Sodingen, Germany (1993)
and the Palais de Justice, Melun (1994), since she set
up on her own.

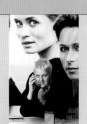

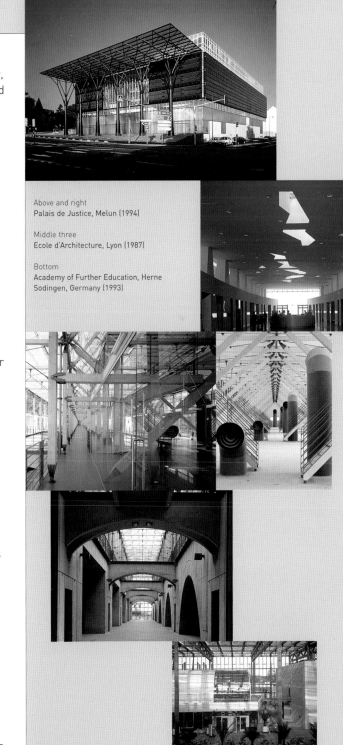

Above and right
Palais de Justice, Melun (1994)

Middle three
Ecole d'Architecture, Lyon (1987)

Bottom
Academy of Further Education, Herne
Sodingen, Germany (1993)

On the other hand, Françoise-Hélène Jourda believes that
'it was easier for me to work without any partner, much easier,
because you just do what you want and I know what I want. And
I'm authoritative'. Jourda has been in independent practice for
about the past five years, following her divorce from Gilles
Perraudin. The law courts at Melun to the south of Paris, and
the widely known Ministry of Interior's training academy in
Herne-Sodingen in Germany number among the high-profile
buildings that, although completed by her, appeared under
the Jourda-Perraudin signature.

The obstacle race began in the classroom. 'When I was
studying' (in Lyon in the late 1970s), Jourda recounts, 'there
were only five women out of 160 students ... and we had a
geometry professor who said, "I know exactly what the results
will be at the end of the year: foreigners will be out, and then
women".' How did she react to that? 'I worked a lot and had
the first prize. It gave me the courage to go further.'

Back in 1985, Gautrand's undergraduate classes were
split down the middle. Nowadays, she teaches at the École
d'Architecture Paris-la-Seine as a third-year projects professor
and estimates that there are a few more women than men.

Eleanor Baxter, a 20-year-old student at Glasgow's
Mackintosh School of Architecture chose Decq's office for
her first placement. At present, 'just under half' at the
Mackintosh school are young women. Baxter reports that
they 'don't feel that they have less chance than men do', and
that 'the numbers are evening out. It can only get more even
from now on,' she adds optimistically. 'It might take some
time but the trend's increasing ... I don't feel disadvantaged
by being female.'

Statistics published last year by the Observatoire de
l'économie de l'architecture du Conseil National de l'Ordre des
Architectes (CNOA) showed that from 1984 to 1997 the number
of female architecture graduates climbed steadily from 29 per
cent to 42.2 per cent. Yet according to 1982 and 1990 census
findings, women accounted for only 7.2 per cent and 18 per
cent of the total number of architects (1999 results are not yet
available). Those registering with the *ordre,* an obligation for
anyone who wishes to build, increased from 7.5 per cent in
1983 to 16 per cent in 1999 – which compares favourably with
last year's 11 per cent on the UK's Architect's Registration
Board (ARB) data base.

So what becomes of the young hopefuls? Do they vanish
entirely from the architectural scene? Difficulties in the big wide

Odile Decq
Since 1998, Odile Decq has been the principal of Decq and Cornette. Works include the Hypertension Intallation for Le Magasin, Grenoble (1993), Banque Populaire de l'Ouest, Rennes, (1996) and buildings for the Université de Nantes.

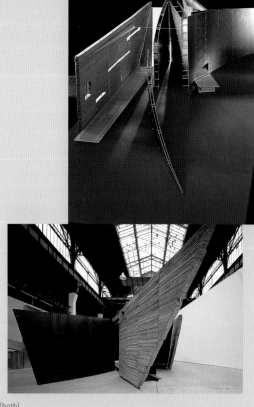

world have apparently precipitated this falling off in the numbers. Social constraints, long hours and the continual battling are just some of the hurdles to overcome. 'You get comments on building sites, which are aspects that men don't get,' says Baxter.

All agree that it is an uphill struggle in the beginning, and Decq is scathing of men that still 'don't know how to answer to us, because [they] don't know how to act with women. Sometimes big bosses don't know how to treat you equally ... I often have people who behave like little boys with me'.

Other pressures on women may also hinder their advancement in the business, such as accepting the conventional role of the mother and housewife. As for children (Jourda has four, Gautrand two) 'nobody can understand that a woman doesn't do the best for them'. An autonomous woman would require a man at home – not easy to find. Even so, relates Jourda, 'in France, it's easier than in Austria or Germany'.

Taxation rules also exacerbate the problem. In southern Germany, Jourda explains, the second income is taxed by 50 per cent, thus diminishing the incentive to work. Baxter wishes to earn 'a reasonable amount of money', so it seems that 'something in property development' is on the cards. In architecture, she says, 'you start earning a reasonable salary when you get to about 45 or 50'. That's too long a wait.

Figures from the CNOA reveal that yearly earnings are, on average, half of what men make. Nicolas Nogue, who collected and analysed the data, questions whether differences in salaries between men and women in society at large are simply reflected in the aggressively masculine construction industry. He also suggests that 'women choose the number of projects and work less because they don't want to devote all their time to [it]'. Going it alone 'is very demanding and women make another choice', such as project management, urban design or generally regularly paid positions in parallel sectors. Overall, they opt for more diversity than men, who elect to follow a more established male role.

What advice would Decq, Gautrand and Jourda give to young women? 'I don't think architecture is especially difficult for women,' says Gautrand. 'We have a lot of freedom.' Referring to other architects, she concludes that 'we are not working in a misogynous environment', and believes that 'there are partners and clients who admire me and are intrigued by the fact that it's me, a woman, who won a competition ... I'm aware of a little admiration'.

Decq echoes Gautrand's sentiments by claiming that 'young women have a lot of possibilities [as] there still aren't many of them, so they're privileged'. She adds, however, that 'it's always difficult being different in a uniform setting, plus, it's a never-ending battle and men are used to fighting'.

'Work', urges Jourda, 'work a lot. Be courageous. Never give up. Work and work and work, and you will win – if you have some talent. That's for [both] women and men.' ⅅ+

Above (both)
Model for the Hypertension installation and shot of it installed at Le Magasin.
Below (both)
Banque Populaire de l'Ouest, Rennes, (1996).

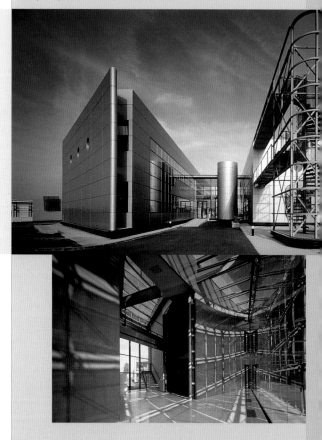

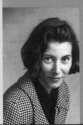

Manuelle Gautrand
Until 6 months ago, Gautrand worked with her
husband Marc Blaising, who ran the management
side of their practice. Works include: Airport Material
Warehouse, Nantes Airport (1996); Secondary School,
Ecully, Lyon (1997); Toll Station, A16 motorway (1998);
the Centre Dramatique National du Nord-Pas-de-
Calais in Béthune (1999); Professional University
Institute, Lieusaint, France (1999); Actair Catering,
Nantes-Atlantique Airport, Bouguenais (1999).

Top two
Centre Dramatique National du Nord-Pas-de-Calais in Béthune (1999).

Bottom three
Airport Material Warehouse, Nantes Airport (1996)

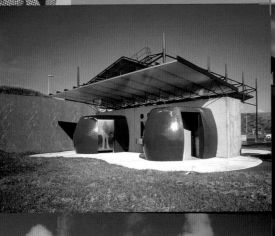

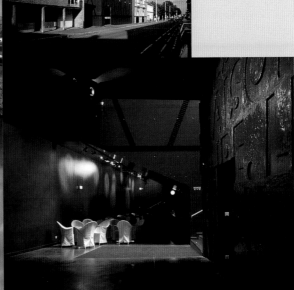

Top, middle and right
Toll Station, A16 motorway (1998)

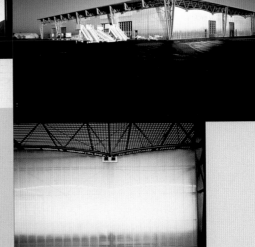

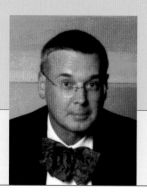
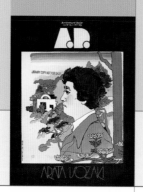

Left
The front cover of the first issue of *Architectural Design* that Haig
Beck compiled as sole editor (no 1, vol 47, 1977). It was devoted
entirely to the work of Arata Isozaki, and included Charles Jencks'
seminal essay 'Isozaki and Radical Eclecticism', which was shortly
followed by *The Language of Post-Modern Architecture*.

Being There

The years between 1975 and 1979 were some of the shakiest in *Architectural Design's* history, with the loss of both the backing of the Standard Catalogue Company and longtime editor Monica Pidgeon. The magazine owed its survival to the staying power of its new young editor, Haig Beck. Here, he recounts how amidst financial and managerial uncertainty, he was still able to deliver some of its strongest thematic titles.

I must have been the only likely person left in London that weekend in 1975 when Monica Pidgeon rang, offering me a position as associate editor of ⊅. I was not yet 30. My experience consisted of making magazines in Australia as a student and a bit more than a year spent as a technical editor on the *Architects' Journal*. Martin Spring, Monica's technical editor, had brought me to her attention, and in the previous few months I'd written a regular column for ⊅. But I was surprised to get the call.

I'd come to London in 1969 hoping to get into the AA Diploma School. In the same week that the AA offered me a place, the AJ offered me a job. Martin Pawley advised taking the AJ position, reasoning that I could always go to the AA later. So I joined the AJ with another cadet technical editor, Peter Davey, now editor of the *Architectural Review*.

As it turned out, Martin was wrong about the secure future of the AA and within a year it looked as though the school would close through lack of government funding, so I left the AJ to attend the AA while it still existed. This was 1971. Alvin Boyarsky had just been elected chairman, and he was to save the school and steer it to the glory in which it still basks today. The AA was fuelled by extremes of ideological and theoretical ferment during the 1970s, and the plurality it fostered has informed my catholic preoccupations as an editor ever since. In 1975, when I received Monica's phone call, the thinking that prevailed at the AA and the networks I had made there would

become crucial to the way I approached editing ⊅.

When I joined ⊅ Monica, Martin Spring and I sat around a vast table in the centre of the big first-floor room of Standard Catalogue's building in Bloomsbury Way, with the art director at the production bench that ran under the south-facing windows. It was a scene of unimaginable chaos: hundreds of files, sheaves of papers, contributors' dog-eared copy, galleys in rolls and strips, and photographs and drawings littering every surface.

Monica tells a story about a visit from the editor of the USSR's Institute of Architects magazine, who had come to London to pay homage to ⊅ (probably the most widely read Western architectural magazine behind the Iron Curtain). He was in shock on seeing the one-room operation that produced this heroic publication, explaining that his magazine enjoyed the amenities of a whole building in the centre of Moscow.

After about six weeks, Monica left to take up a new position as editor of the *RIBA Journal*. Within days of her departure, ⊅ was fighting for its life. Martin and I discovered that the magazine and its staff were to be sold into the equivalence of journalistic slavery to a publishing house with a stable of 30 magazines, the principal one a shoe-making journal. This company intended to rationalise ⊅ down to its two editors.

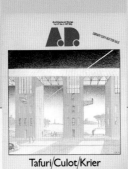

Martin and I walked across to a Soho restaurant to have lunch with the would-be publisher. The night before, in one of the restaurants across the road, three men had been beheaded in a triad assassination. We took it as an omen. When we arrived back at the Δ office in the late afternoon after this depressing lunch, one of the directors of Standard Catalogue dropped in to find out how things had gone. We told him we didn't want to go, and he said, 'Why don't you buy the magazine yourselves?' Standard Catalogue wanted £30,000 for Δ, which at today's prices would be well over £250,000. Martin rode a bicycle and I had a panel van. We looked at him in utter disbelief. But he explained that the turnover in subscriptions was just in excess of 30,000 a year, and that if we paid monthly instalments we could buy the magazine from the cash flow. Standard Catalogue required £30,000 in escrow as a guarantee. So Martin and I set about borrowing £30,000 from his family and the profession, the loans to be repaid at the end of 12 months.

All our efforts went into raising the money. And we also started to think about how to manage the publishing of an architectural magazine, a reasonable question for a pair of novice editors. Martin introduced me to Andreas Papadakis, an experienced publisher and possible third partner. Papadakis proposed that we would all be partners, only he would hold 52 per cent of the shares, and Martin and I would hold the balance between us. Young and idealistic, and bearing in mind his experience, we thought that arrangement reasonable. Papadakis promised to make up any shortfall in the loan we were trying to raise. (I think in the end he lent £2,000 to the enterprise: he got a bargain.)

We raised the money from the profession and agreed to Papadakis's deal, moving Δ to Archigram's old offices in Covent Garden. Δ was Martin and me, a subeditor and a secretary. We designed the page layouts ourselves. Despite this modest office organisation, Papadakis now subjected us to severe belt tightening and we were forced to move again, to Fitzrovia. It was a stressful time, and aggravating the stress was a widening editorial gulf between Martin and me. Martin was deeply committed to sustainability and individual social responsibility, whereas I was much more interested in the new theoretical positions just beginning to appear through the cracks in the supposed monolith of modernism.

The first issue that Martin and I produced together was titled 'Volte Face' (3/76). I sensed that a major paradigm shift was occurring in architecture, away from the model of the architect as social engineer to that of culturally critical practitioner. With this editorial declaration on my part, the rift started to widen. For a year, Martin and I edited alternate issues. At the end of 1976, I took over.

In the Spring of 1977, with the loans to the profession repaid, Papadakis closed down the office in Fitzrovia and bought Martin out. For a few days, I was both editor and part-owner of Δ. But Papadakis summoned me to his office in Kensington and laid down an ultimatum: sign over my Δ shares or be made redundant and lose the shares anyway. If I signed, I was to run the magazine from my home, with no staff and no resources. I wanted to be editor. I signed, packed the magazine production into shoe boxes, took them home and put them under the bed. Each morning, I laid the files on the bed and started work. My partner, Jackie Cooper – who worked at the AA with Dennis Crompton in the Communications Unit – came home every evening and subbed the copy, which was just as well as I couldn't spell then and still can't.

When I took over as sole editor I had the magazine redesigned, keeping Adrian George's familiar logo. We went to glossy paper, abandoning Peter Murray's low-cost alternative newsprint look, and I nailed my editorial colours to the mast(head) with an entire issue devoted to the work of Arata Isozaki (see cover opposite). This was the first shoe box/kitchen table issue. Isozaki's mélange of references and borrowings included Constructivism, Metabolism, the New York Five, Alvar Aalto, the Spaniards, Archigram, Corb and Italian Rationalism. This eclectic modernism intrigued me, so I asked Charles Jencks to write a text to explain Isozaki's position.

The result was his article 'Isozaki and Radical Eclecticism':

architects are once again reviving architectural styles and Isozaki's revivals of the 'New Modern Movement Masters' amount to an eclectic appraisal of the Modern Movement of considerable power. However, unless a theory of Radical Eclecticism is developed, this present revivalist trend will be dissipated too in a 'Battle of the Styles' such as destroyed the Weak Eclecticism of the late nineteenth century and let loose the purist tyrannies of the Modern Movement.[1]

How right he was.
On the basis of this essay, I commissioned Charles to develop this theory and write the first Δ book, its

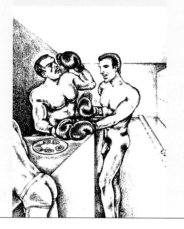
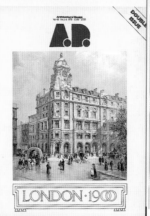
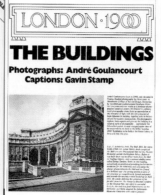
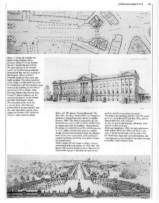

working title 'Radical Eclecticism'. He went off to California and returned a few months later with the completed manuscript: *The Language of Post-Modern Architecture*. The book argued for a theory of radical eclecticism but failed to provide any pertinent example more recent than Gaudí. While this book did not unleash the horrors of Post-Modernism, it provided the textual kernel of the architectural Post-Modernist discourse.

By now, I was 30 and of course knew nothing about architecture. Like the young Ken Frampton, I treated each issue of *AD* as the most stimulating, high-powered seminar from my contributors. Many of the architects who now wrote for *AD* were either AA people or drawn from the AA's stellar visiting lecture programme, much of it directed by the snakeskin-bomber-jacketed Robin Middleton (a former *AD* technical editor). Robin, who was behind some of the best issues of *AD* in the late 1960s, presented *AD* thematics as intellectual and cultural masterworks. In comparison, I felt that I was just playing around.

My second solo issue was devoted to a single building: the Centre Pompidou (*AD* 2/77, probably an architectural publishing first); and aware that no single critique was paramount, I published five critiques of the building as well as three different positions from the architects.

AD 3/77 focused on Tafuri, Maurice Culot and Leon Krier, and included Leo's entry for the original La Villette competition of 1976: it was a didactic polemic positing the reconstruction of the historical European city (see cover and La Villette spread on previous page). One morning, while we were putting the issue together, Leo remarked over coffee: 'I never thought I'd get the opportunity to have my ideas published in English' – an indication of how blighted English-language architectural discourse appeared to the Europeans at the time. Sitting outside ArtNet in Covent Garden with David Dunster at one of Peter Cook's cultural circuses during this period, we were joined by Graham Shane just back from Paris, where, he told us, all the theoretical discussions were about Contextualism. In London we had never heard of it.

AD 5/77 published OMA projects and draft chapters from *Delirious New York* by Rem Koolhaas, an AA contemporary. Ken Frampton, George Baird and Dimitri Porphyrios contributed essays, and I asked Maddie Vriesendorp to produce a graphic representation of Rem's theory of Manhattanism; her response was 'Eating oysters with Boxing Gloves naked on the ninth floor' (fig 3). 'The 20th century in action' is how Rem described it. Before this issue of *AD*, he was barely published.

The young Robert Stern, introduced to me by Alvin, guest-edited 'New American Architecture' (*AD* 6/77), presenting architectural discourse as drawing. The issue looks quaintly dated now, since few of the bright young names of the day are familiar 25 years later. In contrast, the Europeans making their debuts in *AD* would subsequently dominate architectural culture: Rem Koolhaas, Leon Krier, Bernard Tschumi, Antoine Grumbach.

At this stage, I had remarkable editorial freedom. Circulation was rising and I was largely left alone to produce the magazine.

I now switched to double issues, partly a pragmatic decision to catch up on a punishing publishing schedule, but also to gain sufficient space to focus on ideas in much greater depth. An eclectic collection of issues followed over the next couple of years: they included 'Surrealism', 'Bruce Goff', 'Beaux-Arts', 'London 1900', 'Alberti', 'Handbuilt Hornby Island', 'Roma Interrotta'. Most of these themes were on the edge of mainstream architectural thinking, pushing the boundaries of what was admissable to architectural discourse. Previous editors of *AD* had drawn from other disciplines to expand the discourse: social theory and philosophy (Robin Middleton), new technology futures (Peter Murray), alternative technology and sustainability (Martin Spring).

Most of the issues of *AD* produced by me capitalised on events taking place in London. An AA symposium organised by Robin Middleton (a Viollet-le-Duc scholar) prompted the 'Beaux-Arts' issue (*AD* 11–12/78), which brought this arcane architectural period to the notice of a broader and younger readership (see opposite). 'Surrealism' (*AD* 2–3/78) – not an obvious architectural subject – coincided with a major exhibition at the Hayward Gallery. The issue included essays by Dalibor Vesely, Ken Frampton, Bernard Tschumi, George Melly and Roger Cardinal. Gavin Stamp and I dreamed up the 'London 1900' issue (*AD* 5–6/78), celebrating the apotheosis of imperial British architecture – which we were all surrounded by and yet collectively blind to (see above). Bruce Goff inspired an entire issue (*AD* 10/78, see opposite). Europeans then could not entertain Goff as a serious architect: his camp iconoclasm (goose down on the walls, carpet on the roof) made no reference either to the modernist canon

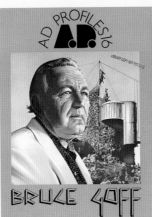

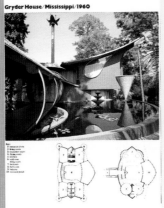

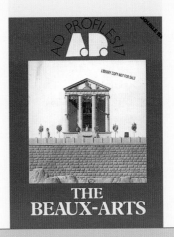

or to an ideological social framework. Yet Goff was one of the most innovative form-givers of the 20th century; and even more significant now is his phenomenological, experiential exploration of architecture. I remember this issue because it was the first time I published working drawings – something that is now the backbone of my current magazine, *UME*. 'Handbuilt Hornby Island' (ᴁ 7/78) featured another territory that was off limits: buildings at the interface between architecture and craft constructed from flotsam and jetsam by owner-builders on an island off the west coast of Canada. 'Roma Interrotta' (ᴁ 3–4/79) was based on an exhibition of contemporary interpretations of Nolli's plan of Rome organised by Portoghesi. It drew English-speaking architects like Michael Graves, James Stirling, Venturi and Rauch, and Colin Rowe into a cohesive dialogue with the Europeans. This issue also included Caroline Constant's map-guide to Mannerist Rome, picking up on an ᴁ map-guide tradition.

By now, ᴁ had been relocated to a tiny, windowless office in Papadakis' headquarters in Holland Street, Kensington. I had been producing theoretical thematics around architectural ideas for almost three years and felt that it was time for a change. Previously, no one in Britain had been building, and consequently there was little new work to publish that corresponded to the new architectural thinking. But things were shifting, and I now wanted to publish projects and buildings. However, Papadakis disagreed. ᴁ's circulation had climbed back up to more than 7,000 and he didn't want to disturb the revenue-producing formula. Eventually, we parted ways after a ludicrous fracas over the cover of the 'Alberti' issue, guest-edited by Joseph Rykwert, which included essays by Hubert Damisch, François Choay and Manfredo Tafuri. On my departure from ᴁ, Jackie Cooper and I started up a new, independent magazine, *International Architect*, focusing on built work. We published this ourselves until returning to Australia in 1986.

Reflecting on the late 1970s at ᴁ, I marvel at my luck in being there. It was a moment when architecture was redefining its thinking and practice, and Britain's pernicious economic recession meant that there was virtually no work, which left architects time to think and write. It was a significant moment and I'm glad I was there. ᴁ+

Haig Beck is a professor at the University of Melbourne. He jointly edits and publishes with Jackie Cooper *ume*, an independent international architectural publication (www.umemagazine.com).

Notes
1. Charles Jencks, 'Isozaki and Radical Eclecticism', ᴁ 1/77, p 42.

Above left to right
'Eating oysters with Boxing Gloves naked on the ninth floor', Maddie Vriesendorp's graphic interpretation of Rem Koolhaas' theory of Manhattanism, as expressed in Delirious New York (ᴁ no 5, vol 47, 1977).

'London 1900' featured a whole catalogue of buildings constructed in London between 1890 and 1914 (ᴁ nos 5–6, vol 48, 1978). The long captions written by Gavin Stamp created a coherent guide to the city at the turn of the century. The title encaptured the current reawakening of interest in Edwardian and Victorian architecture.

Front cover and inside page from the special edition on Bruce Goff (ᴁ no 10, 1978), which gave full coverage to one of the most innovative architects of the 20th century.

Front cover of the 'Beaux-Arts' issue (ᴁ no 11–12, 1978), prompted by an AA symposium organised by Robin Middleton.

Below
Cover of the special issue, 'Leonis Baptiste Alberti' (ᴁ nos 5–6, vol 49, 1979).

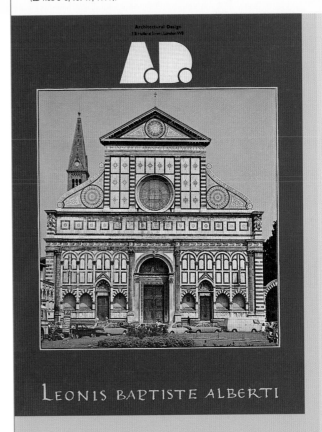

Thomas Deckker:

Two projects in Brasìlia

The British architect Thomas Deckker was offered the unique opportunity of working in the modernist city of Brasìlia, Brazil. Here, he writes about his architectural responses to the city, and the two projects he designed for construction there.

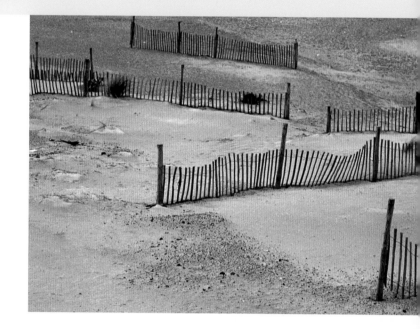

I first visited Brasìlia in 1985, shortly after the deposition of Brazil's military government. At this time, it still seemed that the euphoria that accompanied the return to democracy, and the revival of interest in the great programme of modernisation of 1930–64, might spill over into an enthusiasm for modern architecture.

Brasìlia is the city that comes closest to realising the dream of modern urbanism. It is as distant from its ambitious suburban contemporaries, Canberra or Milton Keynes, as it is from the ubiquitous modern fragments that every European city contains. Although the city was already a historical artefact only 25 years after its inauguration, visiting it made me aware of something beyond the fact that the modern project – both architectural and political – was dead. What was built was certainly courageous and beautiful. What was ignored, however, eventually undermined its foundations, to the extent that the completion of Brasìlia – the symbol of Brazilian modernity – brought 21 years of military dictatorship and the end of modern architecture to Brazil.

What struck me most was the extraordinary amount of leftover space created as a consequence of the design of the city. Some could hardly be missed – such as the huge landscape spaces within the city itself, which resisted the urbanity of the metropolis. Other spaces needed to be sniffed out, such as roofs of the *super-quadras* – the groups of apartment blocks – that were a product of modernist reductivism. These formed uniform platforms six storeys above ground level, usually articulated in each block by three two-storey lift towers.

This roof landscape seemed not only to be architecturally incomplete, but, for me, found an analogous in another very distant and supposedly natural landscape in England – that of Blakeney Point on the north Norfolk coast. There, the shifting sand dunes are propagated and stabilised by rows of wooden stake fences; in other words, the landscape is formed by the architecture. The sand-fences create spaces among and between themselves and the landscape.

Opposite
Sand-fences at Blakeney Point on the
north Norfolk coast. These fences shape
the sand dunes through wind action.

Below
Central hall of the Magalhães House. The wooden wall,
which rises to the central skylight, is cut and folded to
provide almost a 'map' of the house, to give access to the
living room and, upstairs, the master bedroom and study.

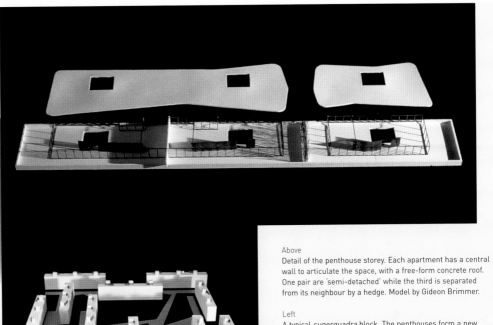

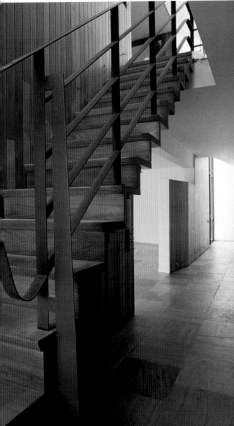

Above
Detail of the penthouse storey. Each apartment has a central
wall to articulate the space, with a free-form concrete roof.
One pair are 'semi-detached' while the third is separated
from its neighbour by a hedge. Model by Gideon Brimmer.

Left
A typical *superquadra* block. The penthouses form a new
inhabited layer. Model by Gideon Brimmer.

Below
A typical *superquadra*. The roofs form an analogous landscape
six storeys above ground. Model by Gideon Brimmer.

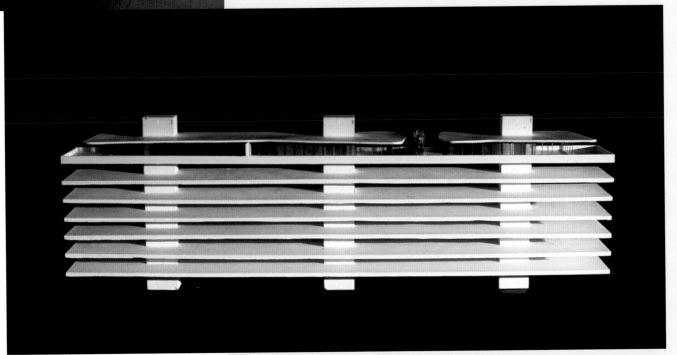

My original brief was the restoration of some apartments in the *superquadras*. To make the roofs inhabitable required only one small addition: a wall placed against each lift tower to define 'front' and 'back', or 'social' and 'service' sides. The single wall in each apartment was intended to be made of the beautiful *sucupira* wood and to be similar to the walls in Oscar Niemeyer's palaces, which play such an important part in the extension of interior space out into the landscape. The only other elements required would be a continuous curtain of lightweight glazing for the external walls and a free-form concrete roof. The sun shines directly overhead, and thus the roofs would cast long shadows down the blocks, out of all proportion to their visibility from the ground.

This project had a political dimension, too. My intention was to add a layer of difference to relieve the social uniformity of the *superquadras* brought about by the sameness of types of inhabitant. Making an inhabitable layer on the top – necessarily for the more sophisticated – was a discerning reflection, I thought, of the occupation of the ground floor by the – unfortunately poor – porters. Just as the domestic space of the apartments is serviced by maids, the urban space of the blocks is necessarily surveyed and controlled by porters.

Next, I was commissioned to design a house in the *lago sul*. This area of the city, bordering the lake, was originally designated for the political class – ministers, diplomats and other officials – but has since expanded exponentially to include the generally wealthy. The ubiquitous 'executive' homes that have cropped up take their inspiration from the incredibly influential TV *novelas* (soap operas), which depict the fantastically exaggerated fictional lives of the super-rich in Sao Paulo. Euphemistically described as 'colonial', these houses are without exception badly planned, dark and stuffy. The starting point for my clients was their wish to eliminate these claustrophobic corridors, which was happily in accord with my own desire to make the centre of the house a space of shifting definition – from entrance hall, to central circulation space, to part of the living room – and to open all rooms off it. The wall on one side is clad with boards of *frejo*, and is cut and folded to provide almost a map of the main spaces of the house. This wall reminded me of a disassembled boat that I had seen in the National Maritime Museum, London, in which the three-dimensional form of the boat was implicit in the spaces between the strakes. The hall is lit and ventilated by a long skylight, which is greatly appreciated by the clients: 'In the morning the sun

scintillates in the skylight and the house lightens as if we were outdoors. At certain times we simply encounter a full moon, exhibiting itself gratuitously'.

Great attention had to be paid to light and view on the narrow suburban site:

There is an integration, almost a continuity, between the interior of the house and the garden. From the study I can see the children playing outside. From any space it is possible to have a view of the sky, stars, moon, sun and garden. It is a wonderful feeling of freedom and well-being …

Two systems of organising spaces are used to bring some sense of order to the house. The first, used in the open-plan spaces, is a series of very large cupboard units used to separate different areas in the living room, study and master bedroom (these are still unfinished). The second, used in the bedrooms on both the larger and smaller sides of the house, is a sequence of cupboard/bathroom/ balcony, which gives each bedroom a secure outdoor space.

To make this house environmentally responsive, virtually all the technologies used in its construction had to be invented or rediscovered. Heavy, insulated construction makes the house cool and calm. Unusually for Brasília, the house has running hot water from a solar-heating system, and the air conditioning is restricted to the master bedroom and study. In the other bedrooms, cross ventilation is facilitated by the traditional *bandeiras* (louvred panels) over the doors. Balconies are protected (against both sun and burglars) by sliding, steel-louvred *brise-soleils*.

Fortunately, all involved overcame the problems of working with an architect based in London, and we were able to achieve an extraordinarily high standard of workmanship. The main part of the house was constructed with a master of works and the finishing stages directly with various contractors. Almost all fittings had to be purpose-made, from windows and doors to the main lighting control panels, and we were fortunate in finding an enthusiastic commitment to the standards required. ⌂+

Both partners in Thomas Deckker Architects are publishing texts on Brazil in September 2000. Thomas Deckker has written a chapter on Brasilia for *The Modern City Revisited*. Zilah Quezado Deckker is the author of *Brazil Built*, on the architecture of the Modern Movement.

Clockwise from top left
The street front of the Magalhães House, Brasìlia, by Thomas
Deckker. The house turns its back on its 'monster' neighbour
while forming an entrance court (and borrowing the landscape)
of its more reasonable neighbour.

Living room of the Magalhães House. The balcony is the clients'
sitting room with access from the study. From here, they have
a view of the garden and pool.

Deckker likens the form of the living-room walls, clad with boards
of *frejo*, to that of a dissembled boat he had seen in the National
Maritime Museum, London.

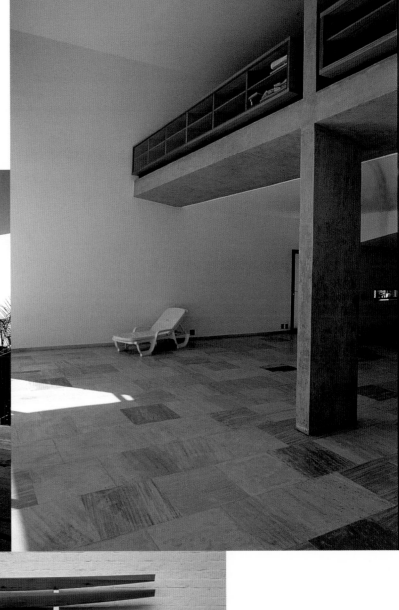

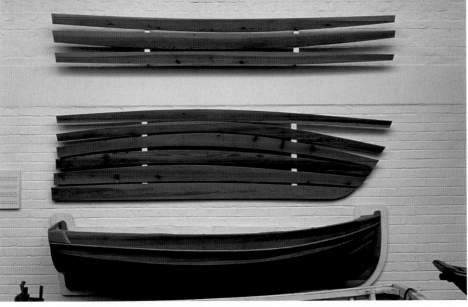

General Lighting & Power

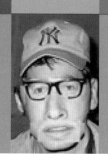

With a name more reminiscent of a utilities company than an architectural practice, it's no surprise that General Lighting & Power has departed from the usual strictures of building design. Iain Borden investigates how this small office, based in east London, pursues its architectural preoccupations through imagery and graphics rather than construction.

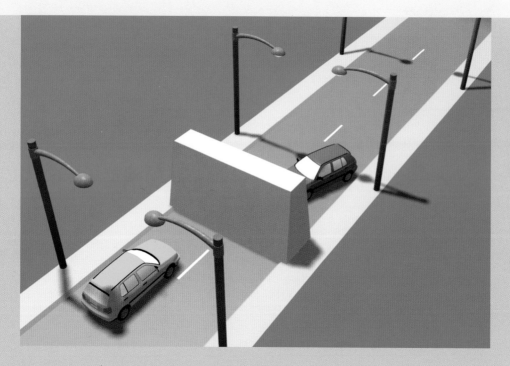

Above
GLP personified. The four members of the practice – Nic Clear, Jonny Halifax, Ezra Holland and Danny Vaia – photomontaged as a composite GLP being.

Left
Highway Code meets *Anarchist Handbook* in the Car Free London project, 1998. Away with the polite bourgeois ideology of new Labour! Car free doesn't mean fewer cars for the masses while the fat cats go around in chauffeur-driven limousines, it means NO F**KING CARS!

Opposite top
Grabs from promo video for Groove Amada track 'I see you Baby' on Zomba Records, Autumn 1998.

Opposite middle
Adidas press advert for Leagas Delaney agency, 1998. One of GLP's 'most architectural drawings'.

Opposite bottom
Car Free London project.

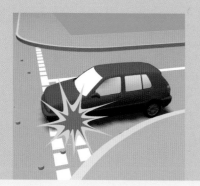

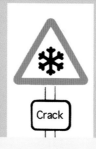

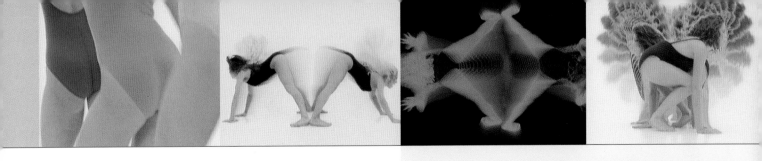

The advertisement features an enormous drawing of an Adidas football boot. It is highly detailed, drawn in the manner of a structure-to-be-demolished, replete with plans and elevations of both boot and goal mouth. The boot itself, according to the hoarding data, belongs to one Paul Ince, of England and Liverpool FC. According to General Lighting & Power, who created the advertisement for the Leagas Delaney agency, 'these are the most architectural drawings we have ever done'. 'Fine', you might think, 'another graphics firm working with architectural conventions.' But General Lighting & Power (GLP) are not graphic designers – at least not by formal education. They were trained as architects, work as architects and even teach as architects. Yet their practice is increasingly being drawn away from the workaday world of schematic design, planning consent, site management and client liaison into another, more fragmented, range of practices. GLP's work is the production of pop videos, adverts, branding and competition designs. And it is still architecture.

Huh? How might the promo video for the Groove Armada track 'I See You Baby' (entirely based around swimwear-clad women performing a sexualised 1980s-style aerobics routine), or a spinning logo (a test for a Channel 4 television brand identity), or a reworking of the Highway Code but without traffic (for the Car Free London project) be considered architecture? What has this got to do with buildings, space and urbanism?

To understand this apparent paradox, meet GLP's four directors: Nic Clear, Jonny Halifax, Ezra Holland and Danny Vaia. They are all 20-and 30-somethings, all male, a bit laddish and, well, eminently likable. Originally, Nic taught the other three when he was a tutor at Kingston University School of Architecture. Ezra and Nic then shared work space together, before forming the practice with Jonny and Danny in December of 1996. Back then, GLP received few commissions, but today things are very different. They work hard. No, they work constantly. They currently operate in that highly fashionable but somewhat down market twilight zone between London's Clerkenwell and Shoreditch: not as far west as established practices like Branson Coates and Zaha Hadid, and not quite as far east as the hip venues like The Foundry, Cantaloupe and Home. GLP command central is above the hyper-trendy magazine *Dazed & Confused*, but you have to navigate blank doors and a blizzard of discarded kebab wrappers to find your way in.

Once inside, the first clues emerge as to what makes GLP and its architecture. Firstly, there's the band thing: the four directors of GLP are like a rock group, which is perhaps no surprise when you discover that their alter-ego band mutation, Fat Midget, sporadically turns out to play to the local art-architecture scene. Like everyone who caught the punk rock/new wave era of the late 1970s and early 1980s, GLP is not afraid to do new things. It made its first promo video not because of corporate strategy or even out of commercial opportunism but simply 'because it was interesting'. Fun, and a healthy disregard for the expert, a willingness to just get up and do it – these are exactly the attitudes that have fuelled a plethora of musical performers from The Damned to The Artful Dodger (another of GLP's new clients). Secondly, there's the student thing: these are also the attitudes of many UK architectural students – particularly those in the London schools – seemingly unfazed by using anything from poetry to resin moulds, Form-Z software to psychogeographic mapping, welding or critical theory. These are the new Y2K Renaissance men and women, able to turn their hands and minds to the full gamut of postmodern opportunities.

It is not, however, just a question of confidence and attitude. It is also a matter of tactics and material. One of GLP's most common tactics is to appropriate architecture designed by others (the Situationist device of *détournement*). Hence, a proposal for a CGI car advertisement includes hard-line perspectives of a building by Holt Hinshaw Pfau Jones. In their poster for the RIBA Architecture Gallery 'Love Architecture' programme, GLP stuffs bits of Giorgio Grassi, Robert Venturi and more HHPJ within a kind of contemporary version of Aldo Rossi's 'Analogical City'. Yet more brazenly, its proposal for the Greenwich Meridian unashamedly sports as its central element the continuous 'worldsheet' surface lifted wholesale from Neil Denari's design for Gallery MA. In the Video Clock Tower project, this worldsheet appears again, flipped on to a vertical axis.

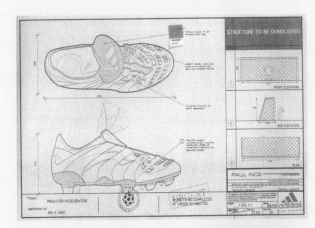

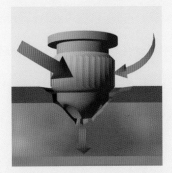

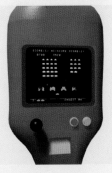

Below
Music promo for 'Let it Ride', Todd Terry on Innocent Records, 1999,
one of GLP's new generation of projects, which are almost exclusively
digital and graphic.

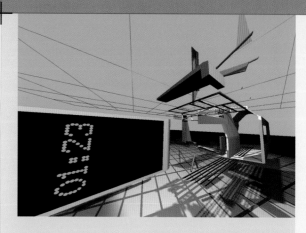

For GLP, these tactics constitute a politics of architecture. It bypasses the production of architecture as finite objects and fastidious details, and goes straight to the impact that design has upon the viewer. So instead of spending years producing hundreds of drawings, in search of a mythic building that may or may not eventually appear, and which may or may not carry a particular meaning to those who experience it, GLP short-circuits the whole process, going straight to architecture-as-image, to architecture-as-effect. Its politics is, then, to be found in the act of *détournement*, and the implicit critique of architecture as an institution that insists on the primacy of the building and the transparency of the drawing in order to achieve its goals.

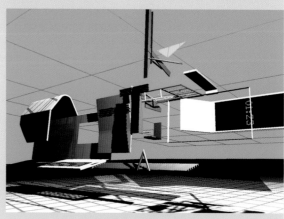

This is also a critique of the role of representation, for GLP's architectural philosophy cannot be 'read' from the final projects. Frustrated by what it sees as the moralising of the left, and by its desire to communicate an authoritative value and meaning, GLP is agnostic if not downright atheist about the possibility of the communication of ideas in architecture. Consequently, if there is meaning in its work, it is to be found in a shuttling of codes and references – what GLP calls the creation of a new syntax – rather than in any referral to distant associations and meanings. In short, meaning is internal not external, performed rather than signed. If, as GLP maintains, architecture is about the creation of urban concepts, while urbanism itself is the way in which we occupy and read cities through our own actions, then GLP architecture is about the creation of cities as a set of informed and critical practices, which take on the full barrage of material accessible within metropolitan life, and make of it what they will.

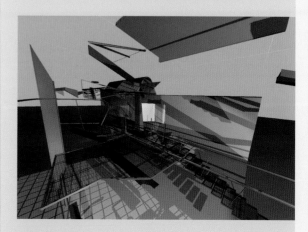

Talking with Nic in GLP's office, it is obvious that it is at a turning point in its development. We sit at a long modernist desk, stylish yet tatty, borrowed from the two fashion designers who sublet part of the floor space. The chairs are not designer items, but seemingly products of the local skip-raiding culture. Yet next door sits a high-end Avid editing suite, while dotted elsewhere are various Apple Macs running Lightwave 3-D with impressive RAM-pumped efficiency. Old commissions for small bookshops (you can see a piece of 'real' GLP architecture in Somerset House) have been almost entirely replaced by digital and graphic projects for clients as diverse as Todd Terry, Nike, KPMG and Peugeot. GLP is also going increasingly up-market – where its early videos tended to be self-produced affairs, nowadays it is represented by the leading agency Bullet. As Nic finally remembers to make that cup of tea, I wonder if many more architectural practices might go this way. After all, it is architecture, just not as we know it. △+

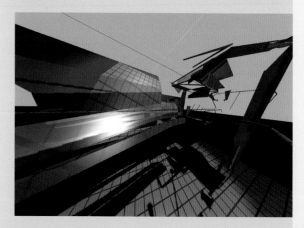

Iain Borden is Reader in Architecture and Urban Culture at the Bartlett, University College London, where he is Director of Architectural History and Theory.

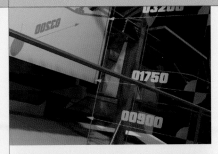

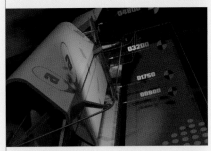

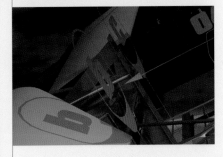

December 1996	General Light & Power Ltd formed by directors Nic Clear, Jonny Halifax, Ezra Holland and Danny Vaia.
Winter 1997	Ideas campaign for XXX-Mas Lights, RIBA *Journal* and Museum of London.
Summer 1997	Music video for 'Disco Machine Gun', Lo-Fidelity, AllStars, Skint Records.
Winter 1998	Invited competition for Greenwich Meridian, Times Newspapers.
Summer 1998	Art direction for Adidas Press Adverts, Leagas Delaney. Nominated for Best Art Direction D&AD Awards 1999.
Spring 1999	Video for 'Let it Ride', Todd Terry, Innocent Records.
Summer 1999	Art direction for Peugeot Poster/Press Campaign, Euro RSCG WNEK Gosper.
Autumn 1999	Video for 'I See You Baby', Groove Armada, Zomba Records.
Winter/spring 1999–2000	Communications Centre for Touchbase Ltd, London.
Winter 2000	Video for 'Movin Too Fast', Artful Dodger.
Summer 2000	Video for 'Nursery Rhymes', Iceberg Slim.
Summer 2000	Advert for CGI, Airbus A3XX, Euro RSCG WNEK Gosper.

This page
GLP's proposal for the Greenwich Meridian Project, 1997, organised by Time Newspapers, who were sponsoring the Meridian Line. The central element is the continuous 'worldsheet' surface lifted from Neil Denari's Gallery MA.

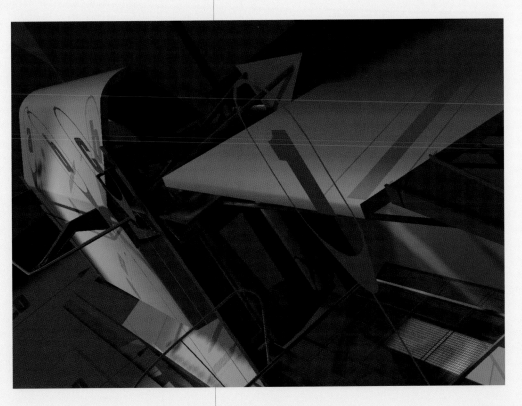

Book Review

Robert Maxwell

Adrian Forty, *Words and Buildings:*
A Vocabulary of Modern Architecture

Thames and Hudson (London), 2000, 339 pages, £28.00.

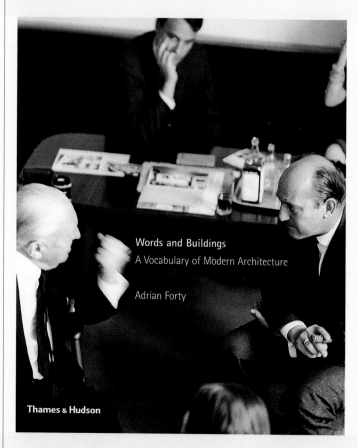

This is an intriguing book, full of magical revelations; at the same time it is mildly disappointing, it raises hopes that it cannot quite fulfil. This is because it carefully avoids imposing a master narrative, which would demand some kind of hierarchical structure, some commitment to an ideal. It deals only with a vocabulary, a sub-set of words, and the structure it imposes is alphabetical; so it's not a bedtime story so much as an occasional dose. This approach may be a useful limitation, a practical way of approaching a subject that is so complex, and full of philosophical and historical questions that have never quite been resolved. It enables the author to cut his way into a dangerous jungle, and on the way to expose a lot of strangely familiar remains.

There is an evident resolve not to exceed the province of factual justification. The author has hung, drawn and quartered his subject so that it cannot rise up and refute him, and so can be conquered piecemeal. The first section has six chapters, each dealing with separate concepts in the argument. The second section has 18 words, each one important in the definition of modernism. Each subdivision creates opportunities, limits the horizon so that the glare is reduced and the detail is exposed. On the way we come upon hundreds of interesting insights, casting new light on a history that we had thought to be exhausted, an implied history of modernism. The well-known texts reappear, but in a new order, and in an unexpected way. The subject is words, the words used by architects and their critics to describe what they do, and to justify it. It is impossible that this subject should not raise very general questions about meaning, in particular the discussion of how words in all aspects of their use are invoked to describe the indescribable, to speak the unspeakable. Like music, architecture is inseparable from the experience of it, and yet it is evident that it has generated innumerable words that are offered as explanation, as justification, as elaboration, as criticism. Indeed, it has little chance of striking home to an individual without words intervening to condition the response.

As Forty points out, words are useful in spite of their inadequacy, indeed because of it. They operate as units in a total system of differences, and this accounts for their flexibility in the face of both ideas and

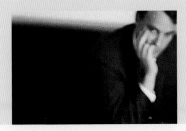

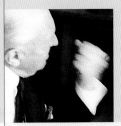

phenomenon. We rush to the dictionary in the course of our arguments to refute our adversaries, but the dictionary is not a directory, like a telephone directory, where names and numbers are irreducibly paired. The meanings given in the dictionary are supplied in the very same words whose meanings we search, the same words merely reordered. It is a circular system. However, words can as well designate abstractions as concrete things, and that is why they constitute such a powerful medium.

There is an interesting thing about the use of words by architects: as architecture became more abstract, in the century of abstract art, it began to benefit more from the abstract aspect of words. This is the key insight of the book, as it sets out to compare past uses of certain words with modern uses of those words. It emerges that there is a vocabulary of modern architecture made of words that have acquired meanings specific to their use by modern architects and critics. The words *space*, *form*, *design* are inseparable from 20th-century architecture, as is the word *function* and its derivatives. Other words like *composition* have almost disappeared from the literature.

The pleasure of reading this book is due to the freshness with which such changes are noticed and elucidated. There is no single chronology, but within each category the chronological history of its evolution is traced, a movement which mirrors and reiterates the broad history of ideas of which it forms a part. The detail is always meticulously exact, but the thought follows a wider and wiser vision that is guided by an overall sense of the cultural horizon. As we find with Samuel Johnson's *Dictionary*, the author's self-limitation to the lexicon of modern architecture does not circumscribe, but serves to illuminate, the steps in the evolution of thought that he selects to deal with.

It is particularly gratifying to find, at last, some recognition within Britain of the power and subtlety of Colin Rowe's criticism. Forty's analysis of Rowe's method (on p 96), which was to focus on the space between lived experience and mental schema, is incisive, and shows how much Rowe was a modernist in his acceptance of the power of abstract forms. In Britain, Rowe's work has, on the whole, evoked a discreet silence. An author who dealt with Le Corbusier and Palladio in the same breath must be suspected of post-modernism, in the particular sense by which most British critics seem to regard that as a contagious disease. Fortunately, Forty is free from the ideological blinkers that have so reduced the scope of critical thinking in this country.

However, by adopting this format, the author does avoid having to create a hierarchy of ideas, or having to erect a structure that would aspire to total explanatory power. The space given to each key word varies, in a way that does not exactly create a hierarchy of importance. This may follow the positive value allowed to accident, or it may conceal personal preferences. One would have expected that the analysis of the word *design*, for example, would have brought in the concept of *industrial design*, and allowed more discussion of the Italian enjoyment of design, relating architecture both to industrial products and the individual lifestyle; a connection that does a lot to explain the character of design in the 50s, before brutalism struck. One would also have liked some more discussion of the relation of verbal theory to visual practice, and some exploration of the steps by which modernism evolved from the white-walled classicism of the 30s through fifties sentimentalism to brutalist realism, from glass curtain walls to historicism, to minimalism, to high-tech and latter-day expressionism. These stylistic vagaries all took place under the supposed theory of functionalism, which says something about the inadequacy of that theory. The importance of abstraction is indeed recognised here, but the relationship between abstraction in language and abstraction in art is not examined very closely. Technology has been a pervasive influence on modern architecture, but it has not removed the drive to create art, so often denied by modern architects, but now acknowledged in the work of architects like Gehry or Libeskind. The great and inescapable discoveries of 20th-century art have been abstract thought (Picasso et al) and conceptual thought (Duchamp). Abstract thought, for Paul Klee, was in principle an approach to objectivity, yet it was in practice a liberation from literality and the rule of *mimesis*, and so a freeing of the artist's subjectivity. How has this paradox affected the evolution of architecture? Questions of this sort remain, there are still questions to be answered; but there is no doubt that this book is an essential step to a more objective evaluation of 20th-century architecture. ⌂+

Canadian architectural writer
Sean Stanwick revisits the site
of a modern classic, the Wandich
Summer Residence by Jim Strasman,
at Stony Lake, near Toronto.

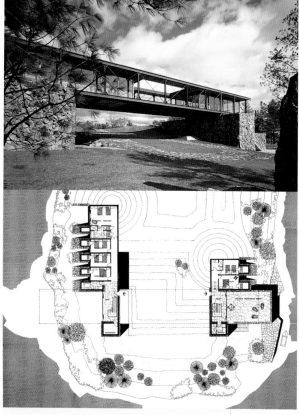

Top
Exterior shot of the house.

Bottom
Ground-floor plan.

At any time in the last few decades, the proposal of a 170-foot steel and glass structure floating 24 feet in the air in the heart of Canadian cottage country was bound raise a few local eyebrows. To do so in 1979, when the glass boxes of the International Style were not held in particularly high regard, may have been biting off more than you could chew. For Toronto architect Jim Strasman, however, the chance to bridge the earth and sky amongst the rugged splendour of the Canadian north was the opportunity of a lifetime.

The spectacular site, a small granite peninsula on the shores of Stony Lake, about 50 miles northeast of Toronto, Canada, is the result of a three-year search by owner Al Wandich, a Toronto developer. The challenge for Strasman, who has worked with renowned Canadian architect Arthur Erickson and is known for his experience in the design of distinctive and dramatic homes, was to incorporate the breathtaking views while minimising the intrusion on the landscape. Strasman reminisces, 'It was such a gorgeous little peninsula that it would have been ludicrous to scatter buildings all over the site. My main problem was to avoid building a camp.' No small feat considering that the programme called for spacious living quarters for five, a separate guest residence and a working boathouse.

Refusing to be swayed by current architectural trends, his solution juxtaposes two opposing paradigms in a tenuous mix of Miesian technological bravura and a site-sensitivity akin to Frank Lloyd Wright. The idea of a bridge structure was not new for Strasman: he has used the form in several other projects. 'I like the drama of it,' he states. Ironically, it was only when wood trusses were eliminated due to size and cost that Strasman realised the transparent qualities of steel and glass: 'Then I began to get excited by it.'

Essentially a giant cantilevered sun deck, the steel bridge embraces the 360-degree panoramic views by adapting a familiar modernist icon: the glass box. The two glass pavilions house the kitchen, dining and daily living activities. But, as Philip Johnson can confirm, life in a glass box can undoubtedly test the limits of one's personal privacy. Responding accordingly, Strasman located the private areas and guesthouse in two granite-clad, earthen berms. As if stepping back in time, the stone ramparts project upwards, like prehistoric mounds of Canadian shield anchoring the bridge to the site. To add natural warmth and texture, Strasman included stone quarried directly from the site, hammered concrete and rough-sawn cedar.

'When Jim proposed the bedrooms be downstairs and the living area upstairs, I was hesitant,' says Wandich. 'But this made perfect sense, because the most spectacular views ought to be from the living areas where we spend most of our leisure hours.' Wandich also worried that the sheer bulk of the structure might impose on the landscape. 'I resisted the idea of steel for some time because I thought it might spoil the look.' Ironically, with almost 7,000 square feet of floor space, it intrudes less on the landscape than the surrounding painted cottages. The lightness of the structure makes it almost invisible, while the use of natural materials ensures continuity with the site.

Without a doubt, the Wandich Summer Residence is as bold and contemporary today as it was 20 years ago. For some, it may seem like an unfinished bridge to nowhere; a well-preserved ruin reminiscent of the great Canadian railways that once unified the nation. For others, the warm glow emanating from the beacon that is a house summons ships as they pass in the night. For Al Wandich, it has become a familiar gathering spot for family and friends in the summer, while a crackling fire provides an intimate shelter safe from an unforgiving Canadian winter. 'Creating this haven', confides Wandich, 'was truly an invigorating process. If I had it to do over again, there's nothing I would change.' ⊅+